Contents

Preface and acknowledgements

'If you really want to know, ask someone who's been there' is certainly true of this book. When we started writing it, we all felt from our experiences of being a doctor, being married to a doctor, being a child of a doctor, or a combination of all three, that we knew all there was to know about surviving in a family with a doctor. However, we also know a lot of doctors, so we decided to ask them and their families for their insights and advice gained over many years of family life.

Throughout the book you will see quotes in boxes followed by names and ages, or sometimes by an anonymous description of the contributor. These have mainly been taken from a survey that we conducted in the summer of 2002 among friends, colleagues and family members who were either the partners/ spouses of doctors or the children of doctors.

It has been very moving to read the honest contributions that have helped us to shape the content of the book. Sometimes we could almost hear the pride, fun and privilege of being in a doctor's family. And sometimes we could hear the frustrations, stress and often hidden pain that this can bring, too.

Some contributors may recognise themselves, while others will find that the 'quotes' are a composite of different people who made similar points. We have tried as far as possible to retain their exact wording as spoken to us or written down in the survey. We wish to thank all of the contributors not only for making the writing of the book so much easier, but also on behalf of the readers who, we hope, will find that your insights and pearls of wisdom will help make theirs a happier and more productive family life.

We are grateful to Professor Brian Jacobs of Staffordshire University for his advice and guidance in relation to the log frame in Chapter 9.

Finally, we want to thank our own families for all of the fun we have had as family groups and the sustained support that they have given us throughout our lives together – the very best prescription for minimising stress in our own lives and helping us to thrive both as individuals and in our careers.

Ruth Chambers
Kay Mohanna
February 2003

SURVIVAL SKILLS FOR DOCTORS AND THEIR FAMILIES

Ruth Chambers
Kay Mohanna
and
Steph Chambers

Radcliffe Medical Press

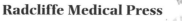

Radcliffe Medical Press Ltd
18 Marcham Road
Abingdon
Oxon OX14 1AA
United Kingdom

www.radcliffe-oxford.com
The Radcliffe Medical Press electronic catalogue and online ordering facility.
Direct sales to anywhere in the world.

British Library Cataloguing in Publication Data

A catalogue record for this book is available from the British Library.

ISBN 1 85775 990 7

Typeset by Advance Typesetting Ltd, Oxfordshire
Printed and bound by TJ International Ltd, Padstow, Cornwall

About the authors

Ruth Chambers has been a GP for more than 20 years. She is married to Chris, a physiotherapist, and has three children, Dave (aged 23), Rob (aged 21) and Steph (aged 16). Her previous experience has encompassed a wide range of research and educational activities, including stress and the health of doctors, the quality of healthcare, healthy working and many other topics.

She is currently a part-time GP and the Professor of Primary Care Development at the School of Health, Staffordshire University. Her doctorate was based on the health and well-being of doctors. Ruth set up a local support scheme for doctors in 1994 and has since run it with the help of other GPs, psychologists, psychiatrists and counsellors.

The warmth and support of Ruth's home life, like that of Kay Mohanna, has sustained her throughout her medical career and allowed her to have a diverse career while her family was growing up.

Kay Mohanna has been a general practitioner for ten years, and is a Senior Lecturer in Medical Education at Staffordshire University. Her teaching interests include medical ethics and epidemiology. She says that most of her insights for this book come from doing the opposite of what she advises others to do here and then suffering the consequences. Her husband is an obstetrician and gynaecologist who, together with Adam (aged 9), Hannah (aged 4) and Maryam (aged 2), has lent wisdom, support and good humour to enable Kay to have a happy family life balancing her GP and academic work, as well as writing of books.

Steph Chambers (aged 16) has opinions on most things. She brings the fresh perspective of a teenager to the problems that beset children who are growing up in a family where at least one of the parents is a practising doctor. Her ideas and critique should provide new insights to help us as doctors to understand the perspectives of our children with regard to the way in which our work impinges on their lives, too. At present Steph is studying for A-levels – in subjects chosen to keep her options open about studying medicine herself at university.

1

Introduction: what's so special about doctors' families?

Why write a book about survival for doctors and their families? Surely modern life places similar stresses and strains on all families in which one or both of the parents have busy professional jobs? Well, while this is true, there are peculiarities about doctors – the type of people they tend to be, and the way in which they are selected and trained, as well as the career paths that they follow – that place particular burdens on them and their families.

Trends in the medical workforce towards early retirement, more flexible jobs and careers and an increasing proportion of women doctors reflect wider societal changes in the UK. However, doctors still seem to have to fit in with a system and culture that makes it difficult for them to have fulfilling professional and personal lives. Many doctors feel that they are expected to give too much of their time to a medical career, to the detriment of their family and personal lives.[1] Consultants commonly complain that their workload far exceeds their contractual commitment to the NHS, and that their current contracts give them insufficient scope for career flexibility and progression.

One study of the relationship between a medical career and family life concluded that 'current Government policies to increase the medical workforce and promote family-friendly policies in the NHS ought to take account of the need for a fundamental change in hospital culture to enable doctors to be more involved in their personal or family life without detriment to their career progress'.[1]

Benefits of a medical career

With regard to pay, doctors are relatively high earners compared with those in other occupations. For example, male doctors in their thirties earn more than 89% of the overall male UK workforce at the same age, and in their forties they earn more than 91% of the overall male workforce.[2] Female doctors are more likely to be working part-time, and a recent survey of GPs showed that a typical female GP earned £32 450 in 2001, representing less than 50% of the annual income of a typical male GP.[3]

Family income was often cited by the children of doctors whom we quizzed as one of the benefits of having a parent who was a doctor. These children often described the material benefits that a doctor's high income had brought for the family (*see* Box 1.1 below).

Box 1.1:

Doctors' families are able to live in larger houses with bigger gardens that are situated in more desirable areas than those of their friends. They are also able to go out to eat more and take more expensive holidays than many other families. These families on the whole live financially comfortable lives.

(Steph, aged 16)

Because of doctors' income, private education is an option for their children, where the other pupils are enthusiastic and children are not stifled by unwilling students. They have opportunities to become involved in more extracurricular activities than students in comprehensive schools can afford. On the whole there is less bullying and teenage pregnancy within private schools. Even though it is hard work and we get more work than people I know at the local schools, I enjoy the atmosphere, as the teachers seem to care about us more. I get to mix with a large variety of people.

(Ann, aged 15)

Overall better grades are achieved in private schools compared to comprehensive schools, which leads to young people having a wider choice for further education for which they are perhaps better prepared and motivated to do well. Motivation to do well, however, may also come from their upbringing, as they have learnt this important characteristic from their doctor–parent, which enables them to apply themselves even better to their schooling. Doing well depends on the attitude of the individual child. These opportunities may lead to a high-powered job with a high income, and a better way of living in the future for them and their own family.

(Matt, aged 16)

I have many opportunities that many other children that I am friends with don't. I am due to go to Australia and the Far East with my school in the very near future, on a netball and hockey tour. This will be the experience of a life-time, and I have heard of no other schools doing anything like this, apart from one other independent school that I only know of as my school plays sport against them in the fixtures that we play on a Saturday.

(Anya, aged 15)

We get to go on holiday to places that none of my friends have visited. I like telling them all about where we go, and they always say that they'd like to go there too, so it makes me happy that I'm so lucky.

(Will, aged 13)

I live in a bigger house than most of my friends, and they always comment on how big it is. I hate it when they call us rich because of it, because I know that my mum works really hard to allow us to live in such a lovely house in a nice area.

(Rob, aged 14)

Emma told us that one of the *benefits* of being a doctor's daughter is their job security (*see* Box 1.2).

Box 1.2:

My best friend's dad has to move around a lot with his job, so she had to move away a couple of years ago and she has moved to two different areas since. I don't like the thought of having to keep moving and changing schools, so I guess that I'm lucky that my dad gets to stay in the same area and in the same job for a long time because of his contract.

(Emma, aged 17)

Sometimes doctor–parents may try to compensate for their absence by being over-generous with money. This can cause problems, as Cath (a doctor's child) describes in Box 1.3.

Box 1.3:

They [doctors' children] are often enabled to indulge in these activities [under-age drinking] due to having more pocket money than other children, and more freedom due to not being monitored because of the long hours worked by their parents. Being given an abundance of money may lead to a depreciation of its value, and they may not be ready to face what financial hardships there could be in the future for them.

(Cath, aged 16)

Why are doctors unhappy?

An editorial that reviewed the reasons for doctors' unhappiness suggested that the following contract should be adopted by doctors and patients.[4] Agreement on these seven statements could be the answer to the most frequent causes of doctors' stress and patients' complaints!

1 Death, sickness and pain are part of life.
2 Medicine has limited powers, particularly to solve social problems, and it is risky.
3 Doctors don't know everything; they need decision-making and psychological support.
4 We're in this together.
5 Patients can't leave problems to doctors.

6   Doctors should be open about their limitations.
7   Politicians should refrain from extravagant promises and concentrate on reality.

The reasons that doctors gave for wanting to retire early or change careers provide another insight into why they are unhappy.[5] Family and personal reasons included the following.

- I hope to spend time with my family as the first call on my attention, rather than with others.
- I would like to enjoy some freedom before I am too old.
- I have given enough to the NHS. I want time to do things which I have been unable to do because of work commitments.
- It's extremely hard work. I can't see myself clinically working at this rate up to 65 years of age.
- I do not feel that I could endure the pace of work for another 15 years.
- The changes in the NHS in the past decade have taken all the fun and enjoyment out of my career.
- There is low morale in the NHS and no one listens to doctors any more.

What do the families think?

The partners* of 18 doctors, some of whom are doctors themselves, completed our questionnaire about living in a family where at least one of the partners is a doctor. We asked them to cite the positive and negative aspects of living with a doctor, and to describe any effects that this might have had on their own career or on the family.

In addition, 13 children (some from the same families and some from others) completed a similar questionnaire.

This was not a scientific research project. It was a survey that we sent to any family, friends and colleagues whom we could think of who might humour us in our search for insight. The sample was therefore selected from people we knew, and just under 50% replied. We were careful not to send the questionnaire to students or others with whom we had any other relationship of dependence that might affect their replies. One of us talked to friends at school, and we all followed up interesting comments with further discussion.

Questionnaires from two of the children were returned with a note from their mothers saying that the children had declined to complete the surveys on the grounds that there was nothing special about having a father as a

---

*Please note that throughout the book the term 'partner' is used interchangeably with 'spouse'. The term 'partner' here always refers to a personal relationship, not to a work context.

doctor compared with any other busy working father. This is a theme to which we shall return again.

Both surveys included plenty of opportunities for people to express free opinions as well as answer the questions. We assured them that their views would be kept anonymous, and that they would only be reported in a non-attributable way. Illustrative quotes are scattered throughout this book, but in addition a brief summary of some of our findings is given below.

Partners of doctors

All of the partners/spouses who replied thought that being a doctor was a good occupation – or at least a mixture of good and bad things. Sometimes this was because of the financial rewards it could bring.

- It provides a good standard of living …
- Having him work, giving us economic stability, gives me the choice to stay at home with the children …
- Job security, good money …
- Little fear of redundancy …
- Because his job is secure, it allows me to be more adventurous in my career …

Being a doctor was also viewed positively because it was seen as a worthwhile or rewarding thing to do.

- It's an occupation with good job satisfaction where one is meeting and dealing with all types of people and it can never be boring.
- It engenders respect and involves the ability to help people.
- It is mentally stimulating.
- It is usually respected by the community.
- Even when he is stressed out, he loves to talk about the job and the people he has met. And when he has a good one [interesting patient] or a 'thank you' he lights up with enthusiasm again. He especially likes the old grannies – I think they remind him of his mum.

There were also other less tangible or obvious benefits.

- It can give a balanced view of life – seeing all types and how others cope. It can be very humbling – when life becomes tough there is always some-one worse off.
- It's very handy to have a patient who is a plumber.

We asked the partners/spouses to list the benefits of their partner being a doctor, and we gave them a list with which to agree or disagree (not everyone ticked all of the boxes).

Table 1.1: Responses from partners/spouses to our survey about the benefits of being married to, or having a partner who is, a doctor ($n = 18$)

Types of benefits of partner being a doctor	Usually	Often	Seldom/Never
He or she takes good medical care of you or others in the family	3	6	9
It has economic advantages – good standard of living for you and others in your family	15	3	0
His or her flexible working arrangements	1	5	12
The status of a doctor within the local community	1	3	6
The status of you and your family within the local community	3	2	8
Remaining in the same area and the same job for a long time	6	2	7
Other comments volunteered about benefits:			
Sharing a common interest (when there are two doctors in the family)			
Educates the children about science and social issues			
Helps the children to think about how they can contribute to society			
Free pens!			

Table 1.2: Responses from partners/spouses to our survey about the negative aspects of being married to, or having a partner who is, a doctor ($n = 18$)

Negative aspects of partner being a doctor	Usually	Often	Seldom/Never
You or others in your family seem less important to your partner than patients do	0	3	15
Your partner does not notice when you or others in your family are ill	0	8	7
Your partner works long hours	15	3	0
Your partner does paperwork until late evening	6	4	7
Your partner seems exhausted even when he or she is not on duty	10	2	4
Your partner has little energy for family activities	7	6	0
Both parents do not attend events at school and elsewhere because of the work commitments of your partner	8	4	1
Social events often have to be cancelled or curtailed at short notice because of your partner's work commitments	2	6	4
You and others in your family avoid socialising or local activities such as shopping because your partner is reluctant to mix with members of the local community, who are also patients	1	4	8
You or others in your family feel isolated from people living nearby because of your different economic position (i.e. you and your family are more wealthy)	1	4	6

continued opposite

Table 1.2:   Continued

Negative aspects of partner being a doctor	Usually	Often	Seldom/Never
You or others in your family feel isolated from other people who try to consult your partner about their medical problems in social settings	1	3	9
You or others in your family are fearful about security at home because your partner is a doctor	1	9	4
You and your family move house frequently because of your partner's job	2	2	7
Other comments volunteered about negative aspects:			
Living in two different parts of the country			
They thought I was a single mum at the clinic because my husband couldn't attend classes for any of my three pregnancies			

Six of these respondents who were partners of doctors were also working full-time, nine were working part-time and three were not working outside the home.

We asked whether having a doctor as a spouse or partner had ever affected the respondent's own career choice. Some of their responses are listed in Box 1.4.

Box 1.4:

When the kids were small I stayed at home because it was hard to share childcare. Even now when they are teenagers, running the home is still chiefly my responsibility.

I am a doctor, too, but I work more hours than my wife. I am aware that it's easier for me – I just come home then go to work, while she has the baby to sort out, too. Her job hasn't affected my career, but mine has affected hers.

It has meant we are limited to jobs in one part of the county. I can't just move around.

Because of the long hours and the responsibility, we felt that we couldn't both be in a job like this and bring up the family.

If I had worked full-time I would never have seen my husband, and childcare was impossible where we lived. Now I could do full-time I don't want to – too old!

I already had a career before meeting my husband, but after marriage and having children I became a 'stay-at-home mom'. It's the children who are the deciding factor in my not working outside the home, but our economic stability because he is a doctor makes it possible for me to stay at home.

I would have liked to stay in hospital medicine, but it's just impossible if you ever want to see each other. General practice was much better for that reason.

With their years of combined experience in adapting to living with a doctor and the demands of a medical career, we thought it likely that these people would have developed strategies that might help and which could be shared with others. So we asked them whether there was anything special that their family had done to make life easier. Their responses are listed in Box 1.5.

Box 1.5:

Regular sit-down discussions, with voting systems for decisions that affect everyone.

We both restrict the number of engagements and out-of-hours activities to allow time for a family life.

We have always had family dinners, and the children have learned not to answer the phone until they left home, in case it was a patient. Paranoia on our part!

Family meals are important to us. We have one weekend a month away from home and the office to catch up with each other and escape the pressures of work.

We make an effort to eat together at least once a week.

I try to deal with all of the post before he sees it. Pay the bills and so on. Otherwise he is on the phone to the gas board, etc., complaining about the bill and getting stressed.

We asked these 'veterans' of the medical marriage or partnership if they had any advice for students or friends' children about choosing medicine as a career. Their responses are listed in Box 1.6.

Box 1.6:

Don't over-commit yourselves and don't have children until you have settled down and finished being a junior doctor.

It's not an easy career. Decide if you are really determined – think long and hard. Lots of time has to be committed, but it is rewarding at the end.

It's rewarding but very difficult, involving compromise and sacrifice of family life.

Go in with your eyes wide open. This may mean considering it as a job like any other, rather than as some mystical job that is respected by all. It is rarely the case, and where it is, 20 years of hard work has been put in already.

I am not that keen that they should, and they know that. But they know they will be supported if they choose to do so.

continued opposite

Investigate different medical roles before making a choice. Don't think that you'll be able to save/change the world.

Go for it – and consider working less than full-time or diversifying in order to recharge your batteries, even if it means earning a bit less.

It's just a job – don't get carried away with too big a sense of duty/obligation. Enjoy its benefits and realise that all demanding jobs have negatives.

It is a very rewarding career – just choose a sympathetic tolerant partner if you choose medicine.

Children of doctors

And what about the children? The offspring of medical parents who were included in our survey ranged in age from 9 years old to adulthood. They had some surprising insights to share. All of them thought that being a doctor was a good job, except for one who cited the long hours as the reason for it not being so. Some of the other reasons were very similar to those given by the partners (i.e. their parents).

- You get all the latest Game Boy games.
- You get to help people – doctors are always needed. You meet lots of people. And the wages are good.
- Lots of reasons – financial, status in the community, rewarding job.
- It's good and you get lots of money, but it could be bad if you don't like blood and sickness.
- I've learned to put others before myself – hearing tales of others' illness put things in perspective.

We asked the 13 children whether they thought that being the child of a doctor had affected their family life. Their responses are listed in Table 1.3.

For those who had not yet chosen a career, we asked them what job they might do when they were older. Their responses are listed in Table 1.4.

Table 1.3: How has being the child of a doctor affected your family life? ($n = 13$)

1	In a good way	6
	(one child said that she thought this was down to the doctor in question)	
2	In a bad way	0
	(even the child who said it was not a good job because of the hours)	
3	A mixture of good and bad	4
4	No different from any other parent's job	3
	(excluding the two non-responders)	

Table 1.4: Careers that children of doctors thought they might opt for themselves ($n = 10$)

Cricket player	1
Doctor	2
Property developer	1
Architect, games designer or author	1
Don't know	5

And what about those three doctors' children who had already chosen a career?

- I became a medical student because I could not think what else to do, but I was actively discouraged by them [the parents].
- Visual design – I'm going to art college.
- I'm a medical student. I think having a GP in the house as a father gave me some insight.

We also asked the doctors' children what advice they would give to other young people who have a doctor as a parent. Their responses are listed in Box 1.7.

Box 1.7:

Don't feel that you're second best because your parent is not there. I always felt enormously proud on prize day, sports day, etc., when my parents couldn't make it, saying that it was because they were doctors.

Make sure they don't work in 'obs and gynae' or family planning.

It can be a bit of pressure in the community, being Dr X's daughter – you always have to be good/respectable.

Don't stress parents out when they come home, as they are very stressed at work.

Make the most of and use all your charms to gain all possible benefits from your parents. However, never ask them for (medical) advice when they have just got in.

Make the most of the hours when they are home.

I don't have any advice. I think every family is different. And if your mother works – it doesn't matter what job she does – she is still not at home.

Don't expect to know whether he'll be home. They have very odd hours.

Get lots of Post-its. You'll need them if you want to talk to them.

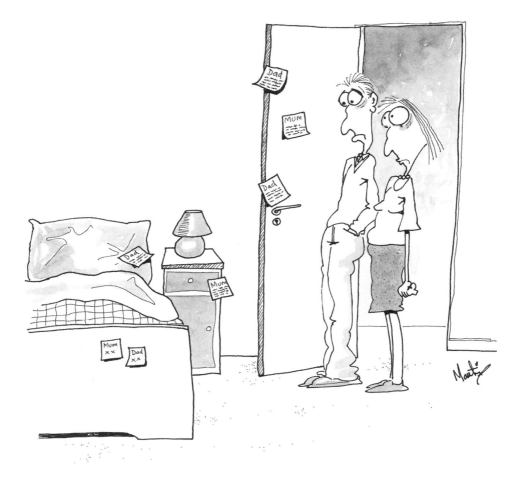

We were touched by some responses and surprised and amused by others. When we asked these questions of our own families we sometimes got answers we did not expect – and not just about career aspirations. Feel free to put some of these questions to your own partner or children, as their answers may be revealing. You can then use their responses for further discussion at home, and you may be surprised where it takes you!

References

1   Dumelow C, Littlejohns P and Griffiths S (2000) Relation between a career and family life for English hospital consultants: qualitative, semi-structured interview study. *BMJ.* **320**: 1437–40.

2   Davies J (2002) *Medical and Dental Workforce Data.* Chamberlain Dunn Associates, London.

3   Smy J (2002) How GPs live. *Doctor*. **27 June**: 51–5.

4   Smith R (2001) Why are doctors so unhappy? *BMJ*. **321**: 1073–4.

5   Davidson J, Lambert T, Parkhouse J *et al.* (2001) Retirement intentions of doctors who qualified in the United Kingdom in 1974: postal questionnaire survey. *J Pub Health*. **23**: 323–8.

2

Career–marriage conflict

Having two working parents generates challenges that are not specific to medicine. The daily plate-spinning act of work, school runs, childcare and out-of-work activities goes on in thousands of homes. These challenges are present even if both partners are working and settled in careers that suit them.

However, there are so many variables in the 'Great NHS Career Structure' that certain specific stressors are thrown into the mix. Married doctors may spend periods apart from their spouse and endure periods of uncertainty and even temporary unemployment that may be unknown to friends in 'civvy street'. Hospital posts, with conflicting on-call rotas and six-month contracts, are not conducive to stable family life or even a long-term relationship, and can cause problems with simple matters such as convincing the bank manager that you are a safe bet for a mortgage.

This chapter considers the career planning of doctors who have partners who also work, especially those who are married to other doctors, and looks specifically at the effects on a marriage or long-term partnership.

Medicine as a career is as popular among sixth-formers as it has ever been. In 2002 there was a total of 11 921 applicants for 6088 medical school places. Some schools received as many as 40–50 applications for each place. However, the BMA cohort studies and other research show that within five years of qualification, 20–25% of doctors will no longer be working for the NHS. This represents a shocking waste of individual talent and resources, not to mention the investment that society makes in producing each doctor. At a personal level it can represent the end of a lifelong dream.

Consider the following mock job description that appeared in the *BMA News* on 27 April 2002.

Wanted: 4500 students with an A and two Bs at A-level to work long hours per week for approximately £5.76 per hour. Ability to make life and death decisions essential. Experience not necessary – full training given (6 years compulsory). Successful candidates will be at high risk of suicide, alcoholism and divorce, but those who persevere may reach top positions after 18–20 years.

In 2001, the General Practitioner Committee of the BMA surveyed GPs' opinions about their chosen career. A total of 23 521 GPs responded, 86% of whom were principals. A staggering 86% of respondents said that work impinged on their quality of life, and 28% of those who responded were contemplating a career change outside general practice.

The relationship between work and family life among hospital consultants, and their attitudes towards the choices and constraints that influence this relationship, have also recently been explored.[1] Three types of relationship between work and family life were identified. They were labelled career 'dominant', career 'segregated' and career 'accommodating'.

- A career-dominant relationship was manifested as a restriction of family or personal life (either intentionally or unintentionally) for the benefit of a career, very often to the regret of those following this path.
- A career-segregated relationship was demonstrated by organised family responsibilities such as domestic help or spousal support, or both, leaving time to devote to career development. Most of the women in this group thought that this was the only way in which they could achieve consultant grade and have a family. However, many of the men in this group were dissatisfied with the balance, due to a perceived lack of choice about the amount of time they could spend at home if they were to be successful.
- A career-accommodating relationship between work and family resulted for women when they took career breaks or worked part-time, and for men when they had restricted work commitments or limited their career goals to benefit their personal lives. Most of the men and women in this group expressed satisfaction with the balance that they had achieved. This category applied to around one in ten men and to a third of women surveyed.

Most consultants had a career-'segregated' relationship, although female consultants were more likely than their male colleagues to have a career-dominant or career-accommodating relationship. Many male consultants and some female consultants expressed considerable dissatisfaction with the balance between their career and family lives. One factor influencing this dissatisfaction was the perceived lack of choice with regard to spending time on their personal or family life, because of the working practice and attitudes within hospital culture, if they wanted a successful career.

There is a discrepancy between young people's perceptions of what a career in medicine will mean to them, and the reality of it as a job. The impact of the reality of the career path for most doctors and their families can come as a shock, as family members describe in Box 2.1.

The presence of two doctors in the same marriage or partnership is a very specific potential source of tension, as all of these factors apply to both partners. A review of GP recruitment issues quotes doctors who feel that their own career has to be put on hold while they are waiting for the uncertainty about their spouse's career to settle (*see* Box 2.2).[2]

Box 2.1:

I thought that one of the good things about being a doctor was that it was a job for life and once you got the job you didn't have to worry about it. I didn't know that when mum and dad got married they had had to move around so much. My dad even went to Scotland for a bit. My mum says it was like being a single mother. I think more people should know about that and then they might not have children until they are settled.

(Sarah, aged 13)

Work as an Accident and Emergency sister was impossible once my husband started work as a GP. On-call commitment for one thing made shift work impossible. I gave up work completely when I had the children – I couldn't combine two jobs – and being a GP's wife is a full-time job. I had to be the stabilising influence in an otherwise chaotic household.

(Ex-nurse, wife of a GP)

Box 2.2:

My husband is looking for registrar jobs in neurology, and as we may be moving I am waiting until he has a registrar rotation before I look for a part-time partnership.

(Female GP locum, graduated in 1993)

Ideally I would like to do a retainer scheme until my husband completes his specialist registrar training. Unfortunately there are only 22 posts in this region and there is already a waiting-list.

(Female doctor on career break, graduated in 1993)

The problems of relocating may fall on one member of the couple, who has to sacrifice their own career for that of their doctor spouse: 'In our three and a half years of marriage we moved house six times. The bulk of this work usually fell to my wife, despite her demanding nursing career ... With our last move my wife could not find a suitable job for her experience and skills, and so settled into being a housewife with all the stresses that "job" implies ... At Christmas my wife said she could not take the situation any more and left.'[3] The strain was compounded by the isolation that this doctor's wife felt because he was studying for higher postgraduate examinations even when he was off duty.

Another problem of location that may occur is for children of a family where the doctor's practice is sited in a rural location or where the parents have voluntarily sought to put a distance between themselves and the patients.

The situation of Eleanor described in Box 2.3 illustrates how frustrating it can be for children in their teenage years to feel socially isolated.

Box 2.3:

Eleanor is 17 years old. She and her family moved out into the country nine years ago. At the time she enjoyed living in the middle of nowhere, as she enjoyed seeing the horses and cows in the nearby fields. However, nowadays she feels very differently, as her social pattern has changed significantly. Now she enjoys going out with her friends in the day and at night, but she finds doing so a lot harder than do many of her mates.

The family had moved after her doctor mother had grown tired of being stopped in the street for a quick diagnosis. She remembers crossing the street on many occasions to avoid patients, when her mum had spotted a patient who was bound to stop her. Eleanor's mother found it too much being continually hassled by patients when she was out, and she wished to be left alone to unwind from work and be with her family in her spare time. She dreaded going to the local supermarket, or taking her children to the park. Even when she was gardening a neighbour would pop her head over the fence and ask if she could just drop round to save having to make an appointment at the surgery. So that's why the family had to move, despite Eleanor and her brothers having friends in their old street.

Eleanor craves independence, but it is simply not possible as none of her friends can drive yet, and because she lives in such a remote area there are no buses to take her to the nearby town. Even though both of her parents work a long way from their house, they still refuse to think about moving as they say they cannot go back to living as they did before, with patients forever hassling them. Eleanor lives a long way from her school, and because of the distance she cannot walk there, so she has to have a lift with one of her parents on their way to work. This means that she arrives a good hour before everyone else, and is picked up an hour later, too. She wishes that the family could move back to the town.

Medicine as a career

Up to now, medicine as a career has had very little in the way of infrastructure or support mechanisms for doctors who are trying to make important decisions about their future. The lack of a clear career structure is a well-recognised cause of stress in any workforce – not just medicine. To gauge the importance of this type of stress in medicine, we have to remember that those who enter medicine as a career were the 'achievers' at school. These were the ones who obtained the top marks in examinations and also had that 'something extra' which convinced interviewing panels that they would make the grade as doctors. After a decade of striving and commitment they enter medical practice to find high service demands and all at once an apparent lack of interest in their career and a dead end in terms of progress and encouragement. They may perceive that there is no incentive to continue their education or personal development and that there are no rewards for further qualifications. If they do still have the drive to pursue extra academic interests and activities, these may have to be fitted in around their heavy service commitments, and will commonly encroach on family or leisure time.

The review of recruitment to general practice mentioned earlier quotes several doctors who were dissatisfied with the level of career support and encouragement that they had received[2] (*see* Box 2.4).

Box 2.4:

I've experienced total apathy and lack of consideration towards me and my career from colleagues in senior posts ... I feel that re-accreditation as a trainer should depend less on local contacts/old boy network and more on audit of trainees after accreditation.[2]

(Male GP, graduated in 1983)

Sometimes doctors end up in specialties that may not have been their chosen career. Many change from a hospital specialty that they would have preferred if they can see that their way to the top will be long or if it is uncertain that it will even be achieved. General practice is perceived by some to be more compatible with family life, and until recently it was not unusual for those who found that their route to the top in hospital medicine was blocked to contemplate a move into the community in search of stability and job satisfaction. However, it takes a certain type of personality to change careers like this and still find personal fulfilment and job satisfaction. Many are likely to end up even more stressed. In a two-doctor family, if one partner has given up their first-choice career for the sake of family stability, this will require an adjustment in priorities and plans that they may have spent many years working towards. If this is perceived as compromise or self-sacrifice rather than as a way of looking after the family or a relationship, it may lead to dissatisfaction and even resentment of the 'successful' partner who managed to continue on their chosen career route.

The review of general practice recruitment[2] quotes doctors who describe such a 'compromise' (*see* Box 2.5).

In our survey of the families of doctors that we undertook in order to gain some insights for writing this book, some respondents took advantage of the anonymity to speak very frankly about some of the decisions they had made (*see* Box 2.6).

Box 2.5:

I enjoyed my [GP] trainee year, but became very disillusioned when unable to get a partnership because of my husband's short contracts. I feel my current clinical assistant jobs are 'dead-end' jobs ... medicine is still very difficult to combine with family commitments, particularly if your spouse is also a medic.

(Female GP, graduated in 1983)

I am bitter that the working conditions in hospital have made me sacrifice a paediatric career so that I can have some time with my family. General practice is much less fulfilling and more boring. However, the better pay and hours make it the only logical choice for many mothers.

(Female flexible SHO, graduated in 1993)

Box 2.6:

If I'm honest, I feel I have failed a bit. I sort of 'settled' for a job in general practice because carrying on as I was would have meant more on-call, and at that stage I couldn't see how it would ever be possible to have a family. My husband was struggling to get to the top in a surgical specialty and I felt I had to move around with him, so a collection of SHO jobs seemed perfect. I went to my school 25-year reunion recently and found myself trotting out the old lines about family medicine being more rewarding, but really I feel I could have done better. I don't really blame him [the husband], but I wish he would stop moaning about how hard his life is – I would have loved his job!

(Female GP)

With all of this uncertainty and potential for conflict, it is amazing that career counselling for doctors is virtually non-existent. Many doctors (both junior and established) have no idea where to go to find information on or practical help with, for example, part-time training, changing specialties or retraining for a different medical career.

Every doctor should make time throughout their medical career to review how satisfied they are with the way in which their career is progressing. Career planning is a must at all stages of a medical career, whether for a young, uncertain medical student or doctor, for an established doctor with a whole range of career opportunities and dilemmas, or when thinking about retirement.[4]

Most doctors report that they have not received any careers guidance or career counselling in the past, and that they have ended up in their current specialties without much thought, having followed opportunities as they arose with little forward planning. The type of careers guidance described by the minority of doctors who have received such help in the past has been the 'Be like me' variety, with senior doctors describing their own careers as role models to be followed. All doctors in training are recommended to have regular careers advice and review. However, a national survey of the extent of careers guidance and advice available found that resources for careers guidance, advice and help were patchy, with few junior doctors, GP registrars or established doctors having access to well-informed, impartial careers advisers.[5]

The British Medical Association advocates the setting up of medical careers services that are 'available, accessible, appropriate, accurate, impartial, confidential, performed by people who have been trained to do it, and responsive to culture and gender'.[6]

So where should you go if you have reached a point in your life when some structured careers advice or information might be useful? Most deaneries have either formal or informal sources of information, and that would be the place to start. Specialist Training Committee members in your chosen field, regional advisers or the regional director of general practice education will all be able to guide you towards the most appropriate sources of help. Many areas are now starting to train personnel in the specific skills required to give such careers guidance, as in the West Midlands deanery (*see* Box 2.7).[7]

Box 2.7:   Example of a strategy for establishing careers guidance services in the West Midlands region

A wealth of experience and expertise has been accumulated in the West Midlands by the deanery personnel, from the human resource managers involved in higher specialist and general practice training to the associate deans and director and associate directors of general practice education. There was agreement that this expertise, based on personal skills and knowledge and involvement with trainees seeking guidance or requiring help, should be available to trainees on a more formal basis.[7]

Helping doctors with career planning can be an involved process that requires dedicated time and training. Any system will need regular updating on changes in regulations for training and appointments, in particular to be able to provide effective help for individuals with complex problems, including those arising from disabilities, mental health problems, disenchantment and poor performance. The unique challenges facing doctors from overseas will require specialist information.

It is clear that the existing personnel will not be able to provide all of the requirements of a fully integrated careers service due to their current commitments. In addition, for some people it will be inappropriate due to conflicts of interest because they sit on specialist training committees or interview panels where there is the potential to meet up with trainees whom they have counselled. The question of who should provide the careers services is being addressed, along with other issues, in projects in three pilot districts that have been identified in the West Midlands. Teams in these three areas will compare

continued overleaf

---

the existing career-planning services with different models of service in terms of accessibility, effectiveness and other outcomes.

It is hoped that a model for a career-planning service will emerge out of best practice, and that it will address all of the needs of potential applicants in a structured and well-planned way. This will rationalise provision and enable resources to be identified for development.

Asking for help from the deanery in your area in this way does not mark you out as more vulnerable in any respect, but rather it identifies you as someone who can bring clarity and focus into the way in which they plan their life.[8] Despite this, you may have reservations about expressing your worries or concerns to others whom you know professionally. Whether it is ill founded or not, this perception can be an extra barrier to your asking for help. In this case there are professional careers advice services that can be an alternative source of information. For example, Medical Forum offers independent career guidance and personal development for healthcare professionals, in person by one-to-one contact or small group workshops, or by email coaching.[9] In addition, for those first contemplating medicine as a career, the Medical Careers Advisory Service, which is run by an orthopaedic research fellow at the Royal Free Hampstead NHS Trust, can offer useful insights and information.[10]

Talking about careers

Suppose you have reached a point where your career is not taking the route you had planned, and you have decided to ask for help. How do you know what type of help you need? Career planning makes a distinction between careers information, careers advice or guidance, and career counselling.

To make a rational career choice, you first need to know a great deal about yourself – your strengths and weaknesses, your personal preferences and dislikes – and then the type of work that is a good fit with your personality and nature. *Careers information* will give you the facts about the qualifications and experience that are needed for alternative career pathways and the opportunities that there are for career progression. That is, it consists of written and/or verbal information about career opportunities, including the number and types of posts available at a particular level and in a particular specialty, and details of the qualifications and training necessary. Sources of careers information need to be up to date, complete and accessible.

Careers guidance is more personal and directive, and provides *advice* within the context of the opportunities that are available. It is useful for those who have not made a career decision, or who have decided on their career goal but do not know the best way of achieving it. A person offering careers guidance could help you to take stock of all of the information both about yourself and about the possible careers, and would then help you to look for a match between them.

Career counselling is a more intensive process that requires specialist skills. Ideally, careers counselling builds on careers advice or guidance, appraisal and assessment, and pastoral support. It includes the recognition and analysis of a person's strengths and weaknesses with regard to the available career options. Career counselling involves a facilitatory approach for students or doctors who are uncertain about their career direction, or who have specific career problems, such as those who have a physical disability or other health problem, or whose career is constrained by personal circumstances, or who seem unsuited to their current post. Such a counsellor would require the skills of active listening and empathy and the ability to step back from a problem-solving approach to one of empowering individual doctors to define and solve problems for themselves.

The extent and type of help and support that are needed will depend on individual doctors' personal circumstances. Established doctors who want to change their career direction may require careers information, careers guidance, career counselling or personal counselling, depending on their individual circumstances and how far they have progressed with career planning. Career counselling has the potential to help doctors at all stages of their careers, but it may be particularly important for GP non-principals who are thinking of returning to general practice, for young doctors who want flexible career paths rather than long-term commitments, and for the one-third of pre-registration doctors who do not end up in their first-choice career.

At a workshop that was convened to examine local careers service provision, deanery advisers agreed that a careers counselling service should offer the following (in rank order):[7]

- remedial action for doctors' under-performance
- sources of appropriate support
- facilitation of individual doctors at times of 'crisis'
- personality profiling
- a service that can 'match' careers.

A careers advisory service should:

- provide guidance on career suitability
- be available at set times within the medical training structure
- be offered to all in training
- be available to doctors at all stages of their career.

A careers information service should give information on the following:

- range of jobs available
- qualifications/training required

- regulations
- personal perspectives
- the local competition ratio (i.e. ratio of the number of applicants to the number of medical appointments offered).

It is still unusual for such comprehensive advice to be available, but the situation is improving. If you decide that you might need to use such a service, spend time beforehand identifying what level of service you think you need. Bounce a few ideas off a trusted friend, and make sure that any adviser you turn to knows the capacity in which you are consulting them.

Patterns of medical marriages

Even if you have taken appropriate career advice at an early stage and been successful in a specialty that you really enjoy, other challenging aspects of life as a doctor, or of marriage to a doctor, might need to be addressed. Different personalities will respond to the various stressors in different ways, and part of the art of marriage is to know how best to help your partner to respond in a direction that will decrease the stress.

Wayne and Mary Sotile are researchers who have investigated the pattern of medical marriages in the USA. They have coined labels for seven patterns among couples, each of which shows distinct behaviours and requires specific types of intervention if it should give rise to problems[11] (*see* Box 2.8 below and the more detailed insights that follow on from it).

Box 2.8:   The seven patterns of medical marriages[11]

1   We're a doctor (traditional male doctor and nurturing spouse)
2   Pleasing others even if it kills them (male doctor and high-powered spouse)
3   Pleasing others even if it kills her (female doctor and her husband)
4   Ready, set, go! (dual-doctor couples)
5   Chaotic desperation (when hot reactors kill the love)
6   The island (when cold reactors kill the love)
7   Too mellow to admit it (two high achievers ashamed of their Big Life)

We're a doctor

This might be described as the traditional pattern of a medical marriage, and as such is likely to be found in older relationships. Doctors in these relationships enjoy the freedom to focus their energies fully on pursuing their careers, which very often results in the two partners living separate lives. The highest risk here is settling for a functional relationship of quiet frustration. The wife may become fatigued and resentful of the absent husband, and the doctor may become bored with the dutiful wife. Once it has been recognised for what it is (a challenge in itself), the solution to any difficulties that this poses may be to find ways of bringing some joint activities into the relationship. It will be important to rediscover areas of mutual interest and to spend time on activities that do not exclude one partner.

Pleasing others even if it kills them

Here the caretaker in the relationship is a driven type A woman who is valued as an energetic person who knows how to manage things. She may be combining her career and home life, or she may have chosen to focus on home and family. Either way, the doctor–partner is left to focus on his career and may assume a 'tag-along' role in the marriage. Such a woman may be attracted to a man who has a more laid back attitude and who is not threatened by her powerful approach, so when this works well it can be satisfying for both parties.

The risk is that the woman may become exhausted as she responds to her need to be all things to all people, and the man may feel alienated or at best uninvolved in family decisions. Irritation among family members may begin to replace the applause. One possible solution would be for more joint negotiation of roles in the home, resulting in more shared responsibility. It might ultimately require a shift in the power base of the relationship, but will certainly require the man to show an increased interest and involvement in domestic affairs and the woman to become less of a 'super-spouse'.

Pleasing others even if it kills her

Some female doctors marry men who assume the role of supporter of their wife's career. When this works well a nurturing husband takes pride in the achievements of the doctor–partner and adjusts his own career to accommodate her progress. However, if the woman changes her schedule to work part-time after they become parents the situation can start to become problematic, as the respective roles become more blurred. Some men may become resentful of a spouse who decides not to take on the traditional family role, with ensuing conflict over which career will take priority. Some female doctors may resent the impact that the family is having on their career and retreat by taking on increased responsibility at work. In many ways this is a similar situation to that in the traditional medical marriage, but here it is the husband who chafes at the growing lack of intimacy. This situation will only improve if there is open discussion and clear definition of the roles within the relationship in such a way that the self-esteem issues of both partners are addressed, as described by Rachel in Box 2.9.

Box 2.9:

I was really lucky with my partnership at home that enabled me always to work full-time. For ten years my husband stayed at home with the children while I built up my career and contacts. I could rely on him totally to run things for the family, and increasingly he supported me in my work as well. When I was doing research he would do literature searches for me and help when the computer played up. We knew what he was good at and what I was good at, and we played to our strengths.

(Rachel, medical consultant and academic)

Ready, set, go

When two doctors are in a relationship, it can seem like a race or a competition. They may become a TINS (two incomes, no sex) couple, as two busy medical lives can leave little time to work on the relationship itself. Even without children this can be a testing pattern, as over time the challenges of balancing the two careers take their toll. One or the other member of the couple will make changes to their career plan in order to accommodate their partner, and if such changes are seen as a sacrifice this can lead to further tensions. A period of contract renegotiation will be needed, as described by Anne in Box 2.10.

Box 2.10:

If I had continued to work full-time I would never have seen my husband. I had a rewarding job, but medicine is very difficult, involving sacrifice and compromise of family life. Something had to give. I don't regret it because I felt the practice got more out of me because I was fresher when I was in work, and the children definitely got better value for money from me since I wasn't with them 24 hours a day.

(Anne, part-time GP and wife of a GP)

Chaotic desperation

Sotile and Sotile coined the phrase 'hot reactor' to describe someone with a low threshold for frustration and a tendency to become overexcited and react with anger when things go wrong. Marriage to a calm, tolerant partner may keep this under control, and the household will be organised in such a way as to keep the 'hot reactor' calm. If there are children, the calm partner will coach them to behave so as not to annoy the other parent, who may become alternately frustrated at the opportunities for things to go wrong in the home and guilty about over-reacting. Eventually the calm spouse may become numb in an attempt not to be upset by every outburst.

In March 2002, a Newcastle-upon-Tyne law firm suggested that the courts should recognise the contribution that a GP's spouse makes to running the practice, just by being the wife of a GP partner. Following the award of 40% of the value of a farmer's business to his wife, they suggested that this recognition was far beyond 'reasonable financial requirements' and was similar to that which a financial partner might receive. This reflects a new financial recognition that marital partners contribute to a successful career in ways far and above what was previously believed to be the case.

Many of the family members in our survey had reached a sophisticated level of recognition of this stress in a household, as the quotes in Box 2.11 show.

Box 2.11:

I was the stabilising force in an otherwise chaotic household. If we were not careful, we could end up walking on eggshells trying not to upset him.

(Mother and GP's wife)

Sometimes I think both myself and the kids have to meet him more than half-way, to be exceptionally tolerant and make allowances – just coping with him being a doctor and being fraught and tired the whole time.

(Mother and surgeon's wife)

What advice would I give to other young people who have a doctor as a parent? Don't stress parents out when they get home, because they are very stressed at work. And don't bother to talk to them if you think you might be ill. All she says is 'don't think about it and it will go away'. I suppose she's fed up with all the sick people at work and doesn't want them at home as well.

(Anna, aged 16)

You have to be careful – not to bring up topics that you know will upset him – and try to keep out of his way a bit. It's hard to keep my little sisters quiet, and I always get the blame when they fight.

(Tom, aged 9)

The island

In this relationship it is a 'cold reactor' who eventually stops interacting with his or her loved ones. Very often it is a male doctor who has hardened himself

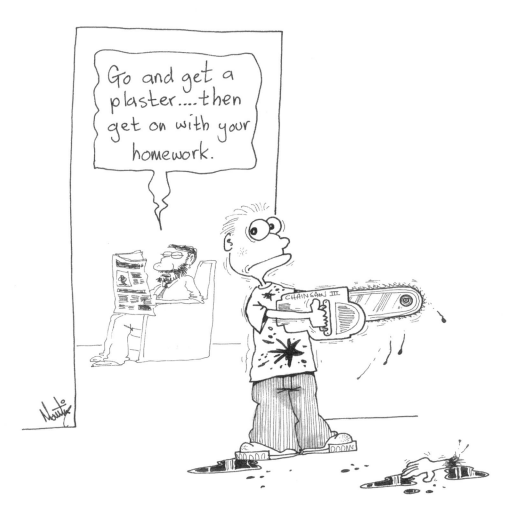

to the stress of a medical life by becoming emotionally distanced. This leads him to appear indifferent to the spouse's life and details of the family and their home life. This worrying scenario can lead to depression in one or both partners. It is difficult to address and may need interventions from outside the relationship, which can be difficult to arrange unless the partners have insight. Agencies such as Relate may be able to help.

Too mellow to admit it

In a surprisingly common modern development in the medical relationship, this pattern affects dual-doctor couples but has more to do with guilt than with achievement and competition between the two doctors. In an attempt to demonstrate their commitment to the modern ideal of life–work balance, both partners try to control their workaholism. The competition arises from trying to manage their type A tendencies which maintain their lifestyle, without letting them take over.

Conclusion

There are many transferable skills involved in being a good doctor that will allow you to address some or all of these types of behaviour. All couples must periodically renegotiate their relationship contracts, and negotiation skills can become finely honed in consultation with patients. The stresses of a demanding job will lead you to develop coping skills for work, and you can draw upon these to help at home, too.

What distinguishes coping, thriving families from the rest is their willingness to tackle unsatisfactory relationships. You should refuse to settle into patterns of life–work imbalance, or to lose sight of the effects that each has on the other. Home is supposed to be a safe haven – a place to return to in order to recharge the batteries.

It is possible to identify the following characteristics of medical families who beat stress together.

- They manage the 'super-couple syndrome'.
- They share responsibility respectfully and fairly.
- They pay attention to parenting.
- They recognise situations and patterns that threaten their relationship, and they do something about them.
- They take responsibility for themselves.
- If necessary they are prepared to seek help.

References and sources of further information

1 Dumelow C, Littlejohns P and Griffiths S (2000) Relation between a career and family life for English hospital consultants: qualitative, semi-structured interview study. *BMJ.* **320**: 1437–40.

2 Evans J, Lambert T and Goldacre M (2002) *GP Recruitment and Retention: a qualitative analysis of doctors' comments about training for and working in general practice.* Occasional Paper 83. Royal College of General Practitioners, London.

3 Diaper C (1992) Life as a junior hospital doctor's spouse. *BMJ.* **305**: 119–20.

4   Chambers R, Mohanna K and Field S (2000) *Options and Opportunities in Medical Careers.* Radcliffe Medical Press, Oxford.

5   Chambers R (1996) *Careers in General Practice: towards a more informed choice. Availability of career guidance for general practice in England and Wales in 1995.* A Royal College of General Practitioners' Revaluing General Practice initiative. Keele University, Stoke-on-Trent.

6   British Medical Association (1996) *Guidelines for the Provision of Careers Services for Doctors.* British Medical Association, London.

7   Harris J and Field S (2001) *West Midlands Regional Educational Strategy Careers Service Pilots.* Postgraduate Medical and Dental Education, West Midlands Regional Office, Birmingham.

8   Mohanna K (2001) Career advice services. *Employ Doctors Dentists.* **38**: 14–15.

9   Medical Forum (contact is Sonia Hutton-Taylor, Director, Greyhound House, 42 George Street, Richmond TW9 1HY); http:fast.to/medical forum

10 Medical Career Advice Service; www.mcas.co.uk

11 Sotile W and Sotile M (2001) Medical couples: the most stressed (and surprised) segment of married couples. *Iowa Med.* **March/April**: 16–19.

3

Team family

Good partnerships with others don't just happen unless you are very lucky – they have to be worked at. In a family, partnerships exist between the adults, between the adults and any children, and between those children. People often utter the slightly tired cliché that a general practice partnership is like a marriage. However, an important difference (other than the obvious one) is that usually in the practice you do work at it. As often as not, relationships within families are left to develop without attention to the bonds between members. It seems more difficult to stand outside a personal relationship and analyse its strengths and weaknesses and consider how things might need to be modified in order to keep it moving and functioning productively.

In Chapter 2 we looked at issues between spouses or partners. In this chapter we shall consider whole family dynamics. Different family members are like different members of a team. Each has a role to play – which may be one they are good at or one that has fallen to them. Behaviours that result from these roles can either smooth the functioning of the family or help to derail it. Personalities, responsibilities and outside commitments mix together to form a heady cocktail that will be different in a partnership that is just starting out to one that is several years and a few children down the line. It is the differing agendas and needs of family members that contribute to patterns of behaviour, and the resulting atmosphere, that form the group dynamics – that is, the interrelationships that occur when groups of individuals work or live together.

Stop and think for a moment. Who is the driving force in your household? For example, how do you decide where you will go on holiday or how you will spend the weekends? Were all of the family members involved the last time you made a major purchase? Who tends to be the problem solver? How do you deal with finances? Are you a democracy or does Mum make all of the decisions? What about fun? Where does that come from in your household? Are all family members involved in their own activities or is there shared time?

Box 3.1 below lists some of the features that can encourage strong and thriving partnerships in which all individuals can flourish and offer each other support. You might want to review yourself and your family against them – just for fun! This is not a scientific test, and you might find yourself saying 'What exactly do they mean by that?' or 'It depends on ...'. It's just to give you something to think about. Score one point for each feature that is present in your partnership at home, and then total them. In a straw poll, we reckon that successful partnerships score about 14-plus.

Box 3.1:   Features that encourage effective partnerships at home (adapted from Chambers and Lucking, 1998)[1]

- The partnership as a whole is greater than the sum of its parts.
- At some point you sat down and thought about where you are and where you are going.
- This dream for the future is regularly reviewed, involving all members.
- The partnership benefits all members.
- There are mutually agreed goals and expected outcomes.
- There are clear roles and responsibilities.
- There is shared decision making on partnership matters.
- Each partner has different attributes that fit well together.
- Members all make a fair investment in the partnership that is proportional to their resources.
- There is a clear commitment to the partnership.
- Joint decisions are implemented by all members.
- You trust each other and are honest with each other.
- All information is shared within the partnership.
- You appreciate, respect and tolerate each other's differences.
- You offer each other mutual support.
- There is flexibility about accommodating each other's needs and views.
- You use language that everyone understands.
- Making the partnership work matters to all members.
- The benefit/burden balance is fair to all members.

All groups have a *centre of power*. In companies it should be the directors, and in families it should be the parents. However, it doesn't always work like that.

We know from our experience at work that poor leadership can lead to poorly motivated staff, aggressive and unsatisfactory interactions, increased time off sick and an overall reduction in morale. The breakup of the team may be the result of poor management, lack of guidance, poor communication and little or no support for individual members or the group as a whole. We witness *games* being played out at work between people as they jostle for position within the hierarchy or try to win recognition and support. Games are often instigated by people to whom retaining power is important, or by individuals who feel that they are powerless.

Similar things happen at home. For instance, what happens when a child within the family becomes the centre of power as a result of bad behaviour, manipulation or attention-seeking behaviour? Or what happens when there are poor or absent leadership figures? What if the family is not a priority or main focus for some of its members? The family can become dysfunctional. It may start to break up, conflicts may arise between members, relationships may come under pressure, and a breeding ground for resentment and general discontent may develop. This in turn leads to factions in the family taking sides, and may result in an eventual breakup.

When this power balance is well managed it can create feelings of security, support and trust and encourage discussion and negotiation, all of which are part of *teambuilding.*

It is unlikely that one member of the family will have been on a 'management course' to help fix things, but you can bring home skills from the workplace that you can apply here. The same dynamics exist, and similar skills can be used to address them.

Individuals within the family who experience difficult times can be helped by applying some of the same tactics you would use when faced with someone at work becoming disruptive or failing to reach their potential. It worked for Susan's family, described in Box 3.2 below.

Box 3.2:

I suppose, like for a lot of people, the children grew up without us noticing almost. Then suddenly there was this great strapping person in the car with me one day saying he was not good at anything, didn't know what to do with his life and could not even decide what options to take at school.

I thought my boy was a confident person, but reassuring him didn't seem to make any difference. I had done an MBA, and it suddenly struck me that an analysis of strengths, weakness, opportunities and threats (SWOT analysis) might help. It didn't cure anything overnight, but I think it helped him to see that I really was interested, and made him actually list all the positives. It's turned into a bit of a family joke now, and when we are faced with a decision to be taken someone will invariably say 'So, what are the opportunities here?'!

(Susan, aged 46, married with two teenage children)

Teambuilding must start at the top. As parents, we need to try to set good examples that will encourage the trust and respect of our children. Without this, no family will be able to function at its full potential. However, trust and respect take time, effort and consistency to develop, and unless existing difficulties are addressed and all family members are committed to the idea of teambuilding, the long-term result may be that nothing will change, just as in the workplace. Equivocal attempts at teambuilding may merely reinforce current tensions and failed relationships. Even worse, if half-hearted attempts at teambuilding are 'seen through' by perceptive family/team members, all credibility will be lost and individuals may feel even less valued.

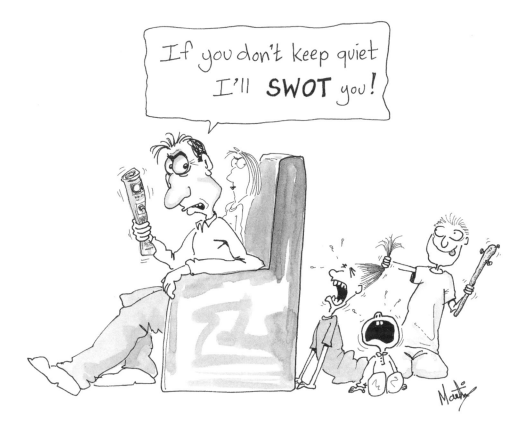

In our discussions with doctors' families it became clear that addressing barriers to good communication was an important issue. This applies not only to the parents, as for any other adult partnership (as was considered in the previous chapter), but also to communication between the parents and children. Avoidance of discussions about sensitive issues is a common and well-meaning attempt to protect children, but may be another cause of poor communication. Children may complain that no one tells them what is going on. If children suspect that something is wrong at home (e.g. the health of a family member, financial difficulties or problems at work), they may come to resent being kept in the dark, or they may feel that they are in some way to blame or responsible for the atmosphere of unhappiness.

It is clearly inappropriate to explain all the ins and outs of an adult problem to young children, but an acknowledgement that there are worries, in a language pitched at their level of understanding, can ensure openness.

Regular meetings where everyone gets together to exchange views become an increasingly important aspect of family life as children get older. The more commitment parents show to family meetings, and the more open the format, the better. There should be opportunities to air grievances in an open forum without others interrupting or being judgemental. Quieter members of the family may need encouragement to speak up. At the very least major decisions such as moving house need to be discussed by everyone, even if the reality is that the decision has to be taken in any case. If this approach is adopted, younger members feel valued and involved, they can say what it is about a proposal that particularly bothers them, and those fears and concerns can then be addressed.

Involving children in decision making may mean that you have to be willing to tolerate the consequences. You need to be realistic about what is on offer in terms of alternatives to be considered. If you truly feel that the route to family openness is to allow them to decorate their bedroom on their own, then all but the most 'hands-off' help with deciding on colours is likely to be met with the response 'But you said I could choose!'.

A similar list can be generated to describe good teamwork in families to that on good partnerships. The list below is adapted from the work of McDerment (1988).[2]

Families that work as a team are characterised by the following:

- agreement about what is important
- openness and confrontation
- support and trust
- co-operation and conflict resolution
- routines and activities that aid communication
- leadership
- regular review
- individual development
- good friendships with each other.

Box 3.3 lists some of the ways in which the families we surveyed talked to and included each other at home.

Box 3.3:
- We try very hard to ensure that we sit down for meals together – not in front of the television. And we always try to talk through and reflect on the day each member of the family has had.
- Try not to isolate children from general practice problems, and always talk through them. Aiming for as normal a life as possible meant that the children were allowed to answer the phone when my wife was on call. This demonstrated that we were a family. However, we did have to have clear guidelines on strategies for phone messages, etc.

continued overleaf

- We had a game at bedtime when our son was younger called *What Did I Do Today?* We would start with 'I got up in the morning and had some corn-flakes', etc. Sometimes he would say things like 'Daddy was a bit sad, so we stayed in the garden.' And then we would know that the atmosphere had got to them a bit. Also it gave us the chance to say 'I was a bit tired today, so I was a bit grumpy.'
- We have a noticeboard at home and leave Post-its on it for each other.
- We always have family holidays that are totally work-free.

An effective team will require a diversity of both skills and roles. Over 20 years ago, Dr Meredith Belbin studied the behaviour of managers who were given a battery of psychometric tests and put into teams of varying composition while they were engaged in a complex management exercise. Their different core personality traits, intellectual styles and behaviours were assessed during the exercise. As time progressed, different clusters of behaviour were identified as underlying the success of the teams.

Belbin's research uncovered nine sets of characteristics that form distinct team roles, and suggested that productive teams have a good mix of roles. You cannot reform your family according to models of team theory of course, but it might help us to explain behaviour patterns within families if we look at the roles that individual members tend to take on. Consider yourself and your loved ones. Can you detect patterns of behaviour in the examples described below that match those which you see at home? Perhaps you can think of ways to incorporate an understanding of preferred behaviours into the way in which you react to each other. We shall return to this later.

Belbin's nine team roles[3]

These are as follows:

- action-oriented roles – Shaper, Implementer and Completer–Finisher
- people-oriented roles – Co-ordinator, Teamworker and Resource Investigator
- cerebral roles – Plant, Monitor–Evaluator and Specialist.

The following descriptions are taken from Belbin's work. They are illustrated in Figure 3.1.

The *Plant* is creative and innovative. These people are responsible for the production of ingenious new ideas and novel strategies. The Plant's preferred approach is to work independently and follow up their own schemes. It may take other members of the team to build on the ideas of a Plant and adapt them to the good of the team.

Belbin team role	Attributes	Allowable weaknesses
PLANT	Creative, imaginative, unorthodox. Solves difficult problems	Ignores incidentals. Too preoccupied to communicate effectively
CO-ORDINATOR	Mature, confident, a good chairperson. Clarifies goals, promotes decision making, delegates well	Can often be seen as manipulative. Offloads personal work
MONITOR–EVALUATOR	Sober, strategic and discerning. Sees all options. Judges accurately	Lacks drive and ability to inspire others
IMPLEMENTER	Disciplined, reliable, conservative and efficient. Turns ideas into practical actions	Somewhat inflexible. Slow to respond to new possibilities
COMPLETER–FINISHER	Painstaking, conscientious, anxious. Searches out errors and omissions. Delivers on time	Inclined to worry unduly. Reluctant to delegate
RESOURCE INVESTIGATOR	Extrovert, enthusiastic, communicative. Explores opportunities. Develops contacts	Over-optimistic. Loses interest once initial enthusiasm has passed
SHAPER	Challenging, dynamic, thrives on pressure. Has drive and courage to overcome obstacles	Prone to provocation. Ruffles people's feelings

continued overleaf

	Co-operative, mild, perceptive and diplomatic. Listens, builds and averts friction	Indecisive in crunch situations
TEAMWORKER		
SPECIALIST	Single-minded, self-starting, dedicated. Provides knowledge and skills in rare supply	Only contributes on a narrow front. Dwells on technicalities

Figure 3.1: Belbin's nine team roles.[3]

Someone who prefers to act as a Plant is easily offended, but responds well to discerning praise. The Plant's behaviour towards other team members can be offhand and critical. However, if they are given space to realise their potential while also controlling their direction so as to avoid the pursuit of fruitless schemes, the benefits can be great.

A *Co-ordinator* will direct the group without being overly assertive, and is able to do this without offending individuals. They are enthusiastic, which helps them to act as a motivator for others.

The Co-ordinator is always prepared to sound out the opinions of other team members, and places an emphasis on communication with others. In general, the Co-ordinator tends to be tolerant and will demonstrate that they have faith in their team members.

The Co-ordinator's enthusiasm tends to be goal orientated. They think positively and, perhaps most importantly, they know how to make the best use of the resources which each of their team members can offer.

The *Resource Investigator* is highly effective when it comes to picking up ideas from others and making them work. They explore beyond the team itself, and have no reservations about probing others for information. The Resource Investigator has strong interpersonal skills. They are sociable and friendly, and are far more extrovert than a typical Plant who is the other half of the team's innovative division.

Whereas the Plant thinks intensely, the Resource Investigator thinks on their feet. Although they are creative, the Plant may not be adaptable, so if their scheme starts to flounder they may not be capable of extricating themselves from the situation. Skilled at negotiation, the Resource Investigator is also adaptable, which may facilitate improvisation and ultimately save the day. Enthusiasm is inclined to flag if the Resource Investigator does not receive stimulation from others.

The *Monitor–Evaluator* has an attitude of detached indifference to the team, and may for the most part take a back-seat role, but will come into prominence when a crucial decision has to be made. It may be that the innovative members of a team will find themselves in debate. The ideas presented by each of them individually may be incompatible, with each advocate being equally committed to his or her own view. A person who is discerning and objective is required to step in, and the Monitor–Evaluator's role is to do just this.

Monitor–Evaluators are very good at weighing up the facts, carefully considering the pros and cons of each option, and finally coming to a well-considered decision. This will be an objective process that is free from the influence of emotional factors. The Monitor–Evaluator shows little enthusiasm or personal commitment; they are not achievers, but their judgement is sound. In many ways the lack of commitment to team goals facilitates the task of the Monitor–Evaluator, because this enables them to be impartial in decision making. Although rather dry and critical, the Monitor–Evaluator fits comfortably into the team, especially if their role is recognised for what it is – both by themselves and by the other team members.

The *Teamworker* is sociable but not dominant. They are good communicators, trusting, sensitive and caring. They will tend to place the group's objectives and the smooth-running maintenance of the group itself before their own personal ambition. The Teamworker is perceptive and diplomatic. They are not critical of other team members, and tend not to make group decisions. The role of the Teamworker is to avert interpersonal problems and so allow each of the team members to contribute effectively. This may be done in a variety of ways – possibly through a good-humoured remark, a word of encouragement, or any form of input which is likely to reduce tension.

Within a family, the Teamworker role of oiling the wheels of team communication may be combined in one person with another goal-oriented role.

The *Completer–Finisher* pays attention to detail. They are hard-working and conscientious, and are good at tying up the loose ends, but they are also an organiser.

The Completer–Finisher tends to be anxious, but their anxiety is not usually apparent to others. Their emotions are generally kept to themselves and they have great self-discipline. The Completer–Finisher tends to work consistently and to aim for success by this means, rather than going for the opportunistic approach with spectacular success in mind. The Completer–Finisher is reluctant to let a matter go unfinished. Although this tenacity is clearly desirable in most circumstances, there are occasions when the Completer–Finisher may hold on for too long, refusing to accept defeat even when a project is not worth pursuing further.

A person like this will be a necessary complement to the more radical team members, who are apt to show great enthusiasm for projects during the early stages of design and planning, but later tend to transfer their enthusiasm elsewhere. The final stages of implementation may be left to a large extent in the reliable hands of the Completer–Finisher.

The *Implementer* is also an essential complement to the team's innovative enthusiasts. The Implementer is conscientious and concerned with detail, and is an excellent implementer of schemes which others have devised. They are also good organisers, capable of directing subordinates, they tend to be well controlled emotionally, and they have a preference for orderliness and routine.

The Implementer differs from the Completer–Finisher in several subtle ways. For example, whereas the Completer–Finisher is driven by anxiety to do the job well and reach completion, the Implementer is not anxious, but is driven instead by their identification with the team together with a set of principles that favour hard work and application. It is because of the Implementer's capacity for application that they are often left to cope with aspects of work which are considered by others to be both difficult and undesirable. Good Implementers are extremely valuable.

The *Shaper* is highly motivated. They have a high degree of nervous energy and a great need for achievement. The Shaper's concern is to win – to reach goals by putting every effort into the process, whatever it takes. They tend to be opportunistic, and will show a strong emotional response to any form of disappointment or frustration.

The Shaper is single-minded and critical, and has few reservations about challenging others, arguing or being critical. At a personal level, the Shaper tends to be an aggressive extrovert, and as such may elicit an aggressive response from other team members. The Shaper may lack the interpersonal under-standing and warmth which are characteristic of the Co-ordinator, and their directive approach is far more orientated towards achieving objectives than towards the stable maintenance of the team. Interestingly, the Shaper's reaction to the aggressive response which they may elicit in others is generally good humoured, as if this is to be expected as part of the process of directing a team.

Since the Shaper's primary role is to inspire action and dispel complacency, their usefulness is extremely limited in a team which is already functioning well and in a stable fashion. In such a situation they may become disruptive.

The *Specialist* is single-minded and dedicated. They are known for their expert knowledge or technical skills. They tend to be introverted, and some-what limited in other areas of performance and group work.

How do the Belbin team roles apply to family teams?

Does your spouse drive you mad with all of the wild and wacky ideas they keep coming up with for family outings or activities? What about the loft extension that they were so keen on last year, but which you were left to sort out when the builders' tools were still lying on the front lawn when winter set in? Perhaps they are a *plant* to your *implementer*?

Maybe that family member who never seems to get stuck in but who always delegates work to others is really a budding *co-ordinator*. Perhaps those skills could be honed so that they can be used to get the most out of other family members. Is there one person who has come to be trusted to have good judgement, but who creates frustration in the others by appearing to be disinterested and lacking in 'oomph'? Perhaps that person is a *monitor–evaluator*. They can be trusted to make decisions at crunch-time, and perhaps you need to learn to play to that strength rather than involve them in projects where their lack of drive and their inability to inspire others will become a real drain on the family.

Perhaps you have a child who is co-operative, mild, perceptive and diplomatic, who listens, builds bridges and averts friction within the family. Is it possible that you have overlooked those *teamworker* skills in your ambition for them to be a dynamic go-getter with exciting ideas for their future? Do you have a *completer–finisher* in the family who is perpetually anxious about achievement and cannot respond well to the *shaper* of the family cracking the whip? Perhaps their slowness is due to over-preoccupation with detail. In this case, is there someone in the family who can help to find a different way to approach things?

You can see that it is possible to start teasing out whether some behaviours can be explained or addressed by attention to the role that each member tends to adopt within the family. Other factors, such as personality and previous experience, will also be affecting this fluid and sophisticated atmosphere that we call the 'family dynamic'. Some psychologists would say that the type of behaviour that it is most useful to understand is the learned behaviour, rather than innate behaviour, since it is the former that is most amenable to change. However, the Belbin approach does give us a framework for looking at how we react to each other and deal with life as a family team.

Perhaps this is something you could talk about at your next family meeting!

References

1   Chambers R and Lucking A (1998) Partners in time? *Br J Health Care Manage.* **4**: 489–91.

2   McDerment L (1988) *Stress Care.* Social Care Association (Education), London.

3   Belbin RM (1991) *Management Teams: why they succeed or fail.* Heinemann, London.

4

Stress and problems arising from stress

Stress is very difficult to define, as it is such a vague word and everyone interprets it differently. Stress is equivalent to a person's perception of the pressure upon them, or the 'three-way relationship between demands on a person, that person's feelings about those demands and their ability to cope with those demands'.[1] In other words, a particular event or task can be very stressful for you on one day but not on another – all depending on how you are feeling and what other pressures are being exerted on you.

Furthermore, what is stressful for *you* might not be so for someone else whose perceptions and ways of coping with pressure are different to yours.

In general, stress occurs in situations where the workload or pressures are high, control over the workload or pressures is limited, and too little support or help is available.

Is stress bad for you?

The answer to this question depends on how much stress you are under, for how long it is applied, and whether you feel powerless to stand up to the stress or you can overcome it. A moderate amount of stress is necessary in order to perform well and to maintain a zest for life. Zero stress may lead to boredom, whereas too much stress over too long a period will render you indecisive, exhausted or burnt out.

Are doctors 'special cases' in suffering from stress?

Stress affects the whole of today's society, and doctors are not unique in reporting escalating levels of stress and low morale. However, in medicine caring for others creates additional stresses due to daily exposure to human distress and ill health, and the urge that many doctors feel to strive for perfection and never make mistakes.

Work-related stress is the second largest category of occupational ill health in industry as a whole, the largest category being musculoskeletal disease. It is estimated that at any one time around half a million people in the UK are suffering from work-related stress at a level that makes them ill. Around 6.5 million working days are lost in the UK per annum due to stress, depression or anxiety, or to a physical condition ascribed to work-related stress. Up to 60% of absenteeism is thought to be due to people suffering from mental or emotional problems. In the UK, 10% of the workforce has been estimated to experience emotional and physical ill health related to occupational stress.[2]

Is stress an integral part of a doctor's job?

It may be an occasional event or task that generates the highest levels of stress, or alternatively more minor but frequent events may cause the most stress. For example, an official complaint by a patient might cause tremendous stress but hopefully rarely happens, whereas inappropriate requests to a doctor to make home visits may be a frequent cause of stress. A steady relentless 'drip, drip, drip' of stress-provoking situations may be just as likely to create a stressed person as a crisis event with monumental stress attached to it.

Box 4.1:

In one study of consultants, patients caused some of the greatest stress in that they were said to be 'increasingly demanding of time and energy, had unrealistic expectations … were increasingly violent and … more and more likely to complain. Complaints took up a lot of time and were often taken very personally by consultants who saw themselves as trying to provide total emotional and practical help "from the heart".'[3]

Surveys of doctors' stress (such as that reported in Box 4.1) describe such a wide range of sources of stress that it seems as if the list of stressors merely represents the ingredients of daily life that make up their job description. In other words, almost everything that doctors do as part of their work has the potential to create stress in some people, depending on the quantity and quality of the sources of pressure and the ability of individuals to cope with or tolerate it.

The types of things that doctors describe most commonly as causing them to feel stressed include the following:

- increased workload
- increased demands from patients
- inappropriate demands from patients

- paperwork
- insufficient time to do justice to the job.[4]

The quotes in Box 4.2 illustrate these sources of stress.

Box 4.2:

The ever increasing shift of workload from secondary to primary care without the shift of personnel or finances, plus the increasing amount of paperwork and computer work, have doubled my working hours in general practice over the past 15 years.

(Female GP principal, graduated in 1974[5])

Increasing out-of-hours commitment is intolerable.

(Male GP, graduated in 1983[5])

Working under the constant threats of complaint (or worse) is demoralising.

(Male GP principal, graduated in 1974[5])

The long hours are very damaging; you tend to fall into a routine of work, eat, sleep, and you become alienated. The rewards to an individual can be tremendous, but at great personal sacrifice in terms of life outside medicine.

(Consultant[6])

It is easy to predict what happens when extra work is continually piled on to an already busy doctor, with too little of the previous work being transferred away and only limited resources available. For a while everything appears to be in order – the doctor keeps going but works a little faster and appears, on the surface, to be coping. However, in order to absorb the additional work, standards may gradually start to slide. There is a conflict between high performance targets and quantity of work on the one hand and professional codes of practice and quality of work on the other. Many doctors put themselves under stress by striving to be perfect and never making mistakes. As quality starts to slip, the doctor may start to take short cuts, fail to do quite what is best for each patient, or treat patients' symptoms at face value instead of exploring the underlying conditions. The doctor may feel guilty and dissatisfied and know that he or she could practise better care. The quotes in Box 4.3 describe the impact of current levels of workload.

The extent to which a doctor is self-critical is a strong predictor of stress. So when doctors are forced to deliver quantity rather than quality and drop their own high standards of care just in order to 'survive', they will be more self-critical and therefore more likely to be stressed.

Change and turmoil have bedevilled the health service for the last decade, as they have done in other professions and services. Health service reorganisations are bound to cause stress because of the uncertainty and extent of change involved, as the doctors' quotes in Box 4.4 demonstrate.

Box 4.3:

My day, to bring in comparable income to the 1990s, is now 7.30a.m. in surgery until leaving at 8.00p.m. I have little family life, no exercise (five years ago I was a keen runner) and am constantly tired.[7]

The only way I have stopped general practice from destroying my home and family life is by going from a full-time to a three-quarter-time principal.[7]

I spend longer and longer in the surgery on a day-to-day basis, trying to cope with the demands that continuing governments create by suggesting that medical care should be available on demand as a right, irrespective of the time of day or day of the week.[7]

Box 4.4:

I am at times very demoralised about how both the Government and the public see/treat GPs and doctors in general. I feel we are very poorly valued both financially and professionally.

(Male GP principal, graduated in 1988[5])

I am disillusioned with general practice. Main problems: (i) unrealistic and often aggressive patient demands; (ii) out-of-hours work; (iii) anxiety over potential patient complaints (none yet!). I work part-time in order to limit/control stress.

(Female GP principal, graduated in 1988[5])

Consultants feel themselves to be squeezed in the middle between the demands of patients, the trust management, the service commitment, the training role, the Royal Colleges and the postgraduate dean's department.[3]

Doctors perceive a decreasing ability to control their working lives due to increased interference by the Government. The research report in Box 4.5 is typical.

Box 4.5:

Consultants complained that important, crucial decisions affecting how, when, where and with whom they were to work were increasingly being made by other people, both inside and outside the workplace. Many of these decisions were eroding their ability to retain professional autonomy even within their clinical practice.[3]

Causes of stress arising from the doctor's family and home life

Stress at work does not happen in a 'vacuum'. Pressures and problems at home often overflow on to how someone feels and performs at work, and the effects of stress at work are often taken home and unfairly dumped there.

Doctors will experience changes and adversity in their lives in the same way as everyone else does. Life events (e.g. marriage, divorce, bereavement, births, etc.) or changes in circumstances (e.g. moving house, switching jobs, retirement) all trigger stress in the doctor, their partner and their family. Some of these life events may come about because of the stresses of a medical career.

Long working hours put pressure on parents who are caring for their children, especially if both parents are doctors, as the report in Box 4.6 illustrates.

Box 4.6:

My 'part-time' full-time job means I work flat out from 8.45a.m. to 3.00p.m., finishing just in time to collect the children from school ... My job is unusual in not involving any on-call – otherwise I could not have considered returning to this level of work, since my husband works long hours as a hospital consultant.

(Female GP principal, graduated in 1983[5])

However, some doctors do get the parenting–work balance right for them, as demonstrated by the respondents cited in Box 4.7.

Box 4.7:

I couldn't spread myself more thinly between work and home. I think I have got the level I wish to have as a consultant, which I can build on, and I've got a wonderful home life.

(Married female consultant surgeon with young children[6])

To cope you need childcare and communication, organisation and planning, and energy to enjoy it. You certainly need a lot of energy, and you've got to want both aspects of life. It's enhanced my life and I'm where I want to be.

(Married female consultant surgeon with older children[6])

Effects of stress on individual doctors at work

Stress often goes undetected or unacknowledged by the sufferer. They may have been warned by others to 'slow down' and have delighted in ignoring such advice and pushing themselves on regardless.

The main effects on individual doctors are symptoms and signs arising from changes in feelings, behaviour, thinking and well-being. The effects of stress impact on all aspects of the doctor's performance at work, and the seriousness of the lapses may vary from slight errors or omissions to potentially fatal mistakes. In the past the medical profession has colluded with managers in 'medicalising' stress. It has traditionally been considered that a doctor who is unable to work because of long-term stress or depression has a primarily medical problem, rather than their illness being blamed on poor management.

The most important consequence of the soaring stress levels in primary care is the high rate of mental health problems and the low morale of doctors and their teams. Studies report that around 50% of doctors (GPs and hospital consultants) may be borderline or cases of anxiety, and about 25% may be borderline or cases of depression.[8,9] By comparison, NHS managers had similar rates of anxiety but significantly lower rates of depression.

The effects of the stress 'virus' on colleagues and staff at work include the following:

- poor team spirit at work
- breakdown in communication
- too little time for each other, so that no deep bonds of friendship or regard are formed and relationships are weakened
- too little support for each other
- others feel stressed when in the company of the stressed health professional
- disruption to new systems if the stressed doctor resists 'change'.

A report of the effects on hospital consultants of prolonged stress due to change described 'evidence of increasing detachment of consultants from their clinical teams as other members developed different roles and working patterns with shorter hours and less continuity than hitherto. This isolation was compounded by fewer opportunities or facilities to meet consultant colleagues, split-site and community working, and a lack of communication or consultation between management and the consultant body.'[3]

The effects of a busy and stressed doctor on those at home

The doctor's relationships with their partner and children are bound to suffer if their energies are completely taken up by work, in the following ways:

* the stressed doctor is preoccupied
* the doctor's partner and children perceive that he or she is disinterested in them, so family bonds deteriorate

- a downward spiral as one problem creates another (marital or relating to the children)
- a lack of support and cohesion
- the partner and children feel that they are unimportant compared with the stressed doctor's work
- potential breakdown of the marital/partner relationship and family unit.

The partner and children of the doctor may be sympathetic to a certain extent, as the poignant quote in Box 4.8 demonstrates.

Box 4.8:

Due to stress at work, my dad has lost all his basic morale and motivation. You can tell when it is at its peak because he spends a lot of time asleep, but still complains of feeling exhausted.

(Vijay, aged 17)

As demonstrated in Box 4.9, a doctor reviewing his career did seem to recognise that his children had missed out on his company.

Box 4.9:

I'm not around as much as I would be if I had another career. My boys have grown up with the situation. If I have not been home I have rung. I would like to spend more time with them, but medicine takes everything except your soul.

(Male psychiatrist, married with children[6])

Solutions to overcoming stress at work as a doctor

Avoid the seven deadly sins of the workaholic.

1. Stop being a perfectionist.
2. Don't judge your mistakes too harshly.
3. Resist the desire to control everything.
4. Learn to decline extra commitments assertively if you are already pressed for time.
5. Look after your personal health and fitness.
6. Allow time for personal growth, the family and leisure.
7. Don't be too proud to ask for help.

There are three types of responses to stress, namely physiological, psychological and behavioural reactions. The way in which you respond will depend on personal factors such as your age, gender, personality and previous family and personal experiences, as well as your coping ability and other organisational options. In a changing world, you need to learn how to cope with stress and its effects in ways that suit your nature. Remember it is not stress itself that is the damaging factor, but rather your inability to cope with it. That way lies survival.

Become more aware of when symptoms of stress occur and how you generally respond to them. Notice what provokes stress in you. Doctors are well known for denying that they themselves suffer stress or other ill-health symptoms, as they perceive such symptoms to be signs of weakness (or sometimes of serious illness or even madness!). So it is important to understand how stress is affecting you, and through you others around you at work and at home, by identifying the sources, effects and consequent outcomes for yourself.

Learn to tackle stresses in your life in a systematic way. You will probably have to learn new skills, such as being more assertive, and controlling your workload so that you can enjoy an out-of-work life. There is a narrow line between behaving in an assertive manner and being aggressive or bossy – sometimes it takes practice to get it right.

Learn to relax so that you can make the most of any free period, even just a few minutes. Try to train yourself to shut right off from your surroundings. You will need a quiet room with no disturbances at the surgery or at home, or even perhaps your car.

Stop being a perfectionist and accept being 'good enough'. Have you considered whether you are setting your personal standards too high and aiming for excellence too much of the time?

Find time for personal and professional development. In order to stay on top, you may need to regain your enthusiasm for learning and your quest for knowledge and understanding. The personal satisfaction that is derived from completing a project, degree course or some other educational experience is likely to make any doctor feel more fulfilled and to reawaken an interest in all aspects of medical practice.

Look after your health. Doctors tend to deny their own needs for rest and recuperation, instead feeling that they are indispensable and playing down their own symptoms of illness. Compare the way in which you behave when you are ill with what most people would do, and try to narrow the gap.

Reduce your commitments. Be sure of your motives for taking on commitments over and above what is required by your main post. If you have just drifted into committee work or felt initially that you couldn't say 'no', this might be the time for you to weigh up whether outside commitments are still worthwhile. Just because you can do something well or find it interesting, or you are flattered to be asked to do it, does not mean that you should take it on when you are already pressed for time or distracted by other pressures.

Six years after qualifying, 8% of doctors who were being followed up in a national survey had taken time out from working in the previous 12 months. Two-thirds of the 35 women and none of the men had opted out of work in order to provide childcare.[10] Some good ways for cutting down working hours are listed in Box 4.10.

Box 4.10:

A study of doctors who had cut down their working hours found that they had done so by four different means:

1   choosing to work less than full-time and/or negotiating to opt out of on-call commitments
2   taking temporary career breaks
3   early retirement
4   leaving the health service to work elsewhere.[5]

A female GP who chose option 1 above said 'I realised I could be a good GP, that my training would be much quicker, I could work in a way to suit me (flexible or part-time), the financial rewards were good, and that I'd have more time and energy for my daughter and for other interests.'[5]

You don't want to end up feeling regretful like the doctor quoted in Box 4.11.

Box 4.11:

It may be that I haven't got the balance right because I'm aware I gave too much to medicine and lost out as a result.
(Divorced childless female consultant in obstetrics and gynaecology[6])

Be prepared to ask for help. Doctors working in a general practice partnership or a hospital department can feel lonely and isolated from colleagues. They may feel that they are expected to keep their anxieties and stresses to themselves rather than burden their colleagues with them. Seeking support is a coping skill that is not often employed by doctors, who may feel that it is a sign of weakness or ignorance. But who will understand your worries about patients' complaints or excessive demands better than your work colleagues? If you express your feelings they may state theirs, too, and together perhaps you can do something about the root causes of your stress.

All types of support are important. The report in Box 4.12 describes the benefits of educational support at work.

Stress-proof yourself by extending your job satisfaction. Job satisfaction helps to *stress-proof* a person and protect them against stress resulting from excessive

---

Box 4.12:

One of the most important factors in reducing stress among hospital doctors in training appears to be consultant supervision. Consultants who sit down with their junior colleagues at the start of a job to discuss educational objectives, offer regular constructive feedback and supervise their clinical practice have trainees who report low levels of stress as well as great satisfaction with their jobs.[3]

---

demands at work. If a person is satisfied with and interested in their job, their motivation will help to keep up their standards of performance and the quality of their work. One of the best ways to stress-proof yourself against the stresses of a job is to explore and expand factors which give you the most job satisfaction. Job satisfaction can be promoted both through continuing professional education and development, and through opportunities for career advancement. If you enjoy your job as a doctor, you feel in control of your everyday work and you find many aspects of the job satisfying, this should minimise the effects of the parts of the job that you find stressful.

We know that GPs are most satisfied by their relationships with colleagues, the amount of responsibility they have and their physical working conditions. One study of GPs found that they were least satisfied with their remuneration and their hours of work.[4] In another study that considered consultants' job satisfaction, consultants rated patient care as the most worthwhile part of their jobs.[3] They liked helping to make people feel better, even if they could not cure them. They valued their autonomy within their clinical role compared with that of individuals in other occupations. Without job satisfaction, stress is more likely to creep in.

Studies of job satisfaction in organisations in general show that employees rate achievement, recognition, responsibility, advancement and growth more highly than salary, status, security, supervision, relationships with work colleagues and working conditions. A study of young people's work ethic found that 'Generation X' (the 18–29 years age group) wants stimulating work, variety, to be constantly learning and to receive continuous feedback on how they are doing.[11]

Build strong, mutually supportive networks with other colleagues at work. We know from research on stress that individuals with the best social supports who interact well with other people have the greatest ability to cope with stress, and are the least affected by it.

Effective partnerships in general practice have been shown to help individual GPs to combat low morale and manage their workload. Building and maintaining strong and supportive partnerships needs protected time for the GP partners and practice staff to get together, as well as some slack in their daily work routines to allow 'personal and group problems to be noticed and tackled proactively, rather than reactively'.[12]

Consider some tips for your happiness at work. A recent newspaper article recommended the following ten actions that people can take in order to be more happy with their work.[13]

1   Define your own idea of success at work, and then stick to that and not to other people's definitions.
2   Avoid 'hurry-sickness' by allocating realistic amounts of time for achieving your most important tasks.
3   Don't be anxious – be happy. Do something about the causes of your anxiety as far as you can.
4   Beware of the activity trap – resist becoming addicted to constant activity.
5   Don't burn out – create a health plan.
6   Switch off – separate work from the rest of your life.
7   Watch out for 'false success' – don't confuse success with endless activity.
8   Manage urgency by prioritising tasks according to their importance rather than their urgency.
9   Give up struggling – find a better way to do things more easily, and don't battle with stress and work overload.
10   Bring the fun back into your working life and that of your team.

Overcoming stress at home for doctors and their families

No family is immune from the pressures of modern life, and medical families have all of the ingredients for fallout and breakdown.

But how do we know that the stresses which impact on a doctor's family do so solely because of the commitments of that occupation? Is stress in doctors' families due to the lifestyle that is brought about by at least one parent being a doctor? Or is it because a certain sort of person is drawn to a career as a doctor, and doctors have a different outlook to most of the rest of the general population with regard to how to bring up their families? Many of the children whom we interviewed reported that their doctor–parent had said that if they could have their time all over again, they would definitely not be a doctor. Two quotes from doctors' children about the perceived negative effects of the doctor on family life are cited in Box 4.13.

Box 4.13:

A doctor's family is subjected to grumbles about the doctor's unreasonable hours, their misuse by the Government/NHS, pointless waiting-list initiatives, restrictions on life-saving drugs because of their expense ... the list is never-ending.

(Cath, aged 16)

When asked by my mum what my two brothers and I were considering being when we were older, none of us really knew or had thought about it that deeply. However, what we were adamant about was that we were definitely *not* going to be doctors, and we still all hold that view. I think that is because we have only been subjected to the negativities of the job. We don't know when our mum has had a good day, just a bad one. We have noticed her absence when she has been on call throughout Christmas, when she'd had to dash out between opening presents and pulling crackers. I could not name five enjoyable things that she experiences at work, but I could name 50 aspects that she hates.

(Tom, aged 14)

Developing supportive relationships at home

If you have a close and supportive partner and family at home, that will be a good safe place to offload and share your worries about work, so long as this does not strain your relationship unduly. However, many doctors do not have such a close personal relationship with a partner, as being single or divorced is common among doctors, and they may have few friends outside work if they have let their workaholic and medicine-centred interests dominate their lives.

Communication

If tensions within the family are getting out of hand, the priority is to re-establish better communication, whatever the causes. The first step may be to try to distance yourself from your feelings about the situation and look at it from a different viewpoint.

Whole family approach. Call a family meeting and let everyone have a chance to air their grievances or offer their ideas. Family members need to feel safe enough to speak honestly, but don't have too high expectations at first, as they may need time and space to express themselves. This is not a 10-minute consultation, and it is important for you as a parent to get out of the doctor role and become an ordinary family member with good listening skills.

Family priorities. Regularly re-evaluate those extra commitments that are keeping you away from the family, especially in the evenings and at weekends, and see if there are any that you might drop. Do not regard this as self-sacrifice, but as something that you are doing as part of looking after yourself and your family. Get work-related worries off your chest when you come home, and then put them aside.

Take time out. Take regular holidays, and if you and your colleagues provide cover for each other for holidays and courses, try to persuade others at work to employ locums in future. The improved quality of life may justify the expense or loss of income – ask the family!

Building fulfilment in your family life

Maslow has described how self-esteem and fulfilment are not possible if the basic structure and safety components of your life are not secure.[14] Self-esteem encompassing self-respect, status and recognition from others is only possible if it is built upon a good social base that includes love, friendship, belonging to groups (work, home, leisure, professional) and social activities. Fulfilment, maturity and wisdom are only possible if all of the other conditions of a person's life encourage growth, personal development and accomplishment.

One of the ingredients for a secure base is time for family life (not perceived by the doctor cited in Box 4.14 to be available to those with a full-time medical career).

Box 4.14:

The increasingly unreasonable demands of patients and abuse of the GPs' system are largely responsible for this career being incompatible with a family lifestyle, without complete neglect of my own personal and family needs.

(Male doctor, graduated in 1988[5])

Negotiating decisions that affect your life

If you decide that the shape of your working week needs an overhaul, you will need to negotiate that change with others.

Negotiating is an integral part of assertive behaviour that is used to reach a mutually acceptable agreement which suits both parties. For instance, you might need to negotiate with your partner or spouse about whose career is going to take precedence at various stages of your lives together. Prepare your arguments well using logic based on facts and figures, rather than offering veiled threats or empty promises. Give a fair assessment of the current situation, without exaggerating or minimising the problems, issues or challenges involved. You will need to be clear about your objectives in any negotiations. State your most important requirements clearly in a straightforward manner, and describe the benefits for the other person.

Listen carefully to the other person's viewpoint so that you can understand their position and concerns. Clarify what they are saying and their position and the exact terms and conditions they are offering. Summarise what you think they have just said in order to check the wording and ensure that there are no ambiguities. Ask open questions to obtain information, and find out what their 'bottom line' is, as well as looking for weaknesses or unfairness in their arguments.

Avoid confrontation or a stalemate by offering other options which you have worked out beforehand as being acceptable alternative solutions. Discuss how you each might trade concessions so as to reach an acceptable agreement. If the other person makes a concession, don't gloat. It is important to avoid loss of face for either party if the negotiations are to remain amicable. Give the other person time to reflect on your request and work through your suggested ideas or changes, rather than demanding an instant response. Once you have reached agreement, close the discussion. Ruminating on the problems or different options will only waste time, and the other party may try to reopen negotiations or backtrack on your agreement.

The quotes in Box 4.15 describe the career decisions that individuals negotiated with their partners, some more willingly than others.

Box 4.15:

I had always been quite interested in general practice, and my partner's decision to opt for a hospital career meant that I could be more mobile to follow her as a GP.

(Male career break/locum, graduated in 1993[5])

I left my post as a partner in general practice two months ago after 18 years in the practice. I left to accompany my husband on a two-year posting abroad. Now I'm a locum on a military base. I work as GP/casualty officer.

(Female locum, graduated in 1974[5])

Working child-friendly hours

Some medical specialties are appreciated by young doctors for their potential flexibility in fitting around the family's needs. However, this can have its downside, too, in leading to a less fulfilling post, according to one of the doctors cited in Box 4.16.

> **Box 4.16:**   Doctors who have changed career direction in order to accommodate their families' needs
>
> General practice has good flexibility (i.e. I can choose exactly the amount of sessions I wish to work as a GP and can easily find a job in the local area – this all fits in well with my childcare commitments).
>
>   (Female doctor, qualified 6 years previously[10])
>
> I continue to find it very hard balancing career with family life. However, my present job has been created to fit in with school hours, which is excellent. The downside is that my job is very quiet and on the research/outpatient side of medicine, and not very fulfilling.
>
>   (Female doctor[10])

There are schemes that enable doctors to work in a limited part-time way as part of a 'career break' to 'keep their hand in' while their children are young. The NHS Flexible Careers Scheme has been designed so that a senior house officer or specialist registrar works a minimum of two sessions a week, up to a maximum of 49% of the working week. The doctor can then resume their training at the end of their 'break'. This scheme has been extended to include GPs. The general practitioner retainer scheme allows a GP to work up to four sessions a week.

Skills that doctors and their families should learn

Relaxation for stress relief

Find the method that works best for you. Some people find hard exercise more beneficial than deep relaxation. Why not buy or borrow a relaxation tape and see if it is helpful for you? Choose a time when, and place where, you are unlikely to be disturbed, lie back in an armchair or stretch out on a comfortable bed, and play the tape through twice. If you are someone who finds it difficult to relax, and who becomes fidgety if they are waiting around with nothing to do, you will find that you have to be very firm with yourself about listening quietly to the relaxation sessions.

Increase your motivation

Different people are motivated by different things, and arguments rage as to whether anyone is ever driven by entirely altruistic motives. Obviously money motivates some individuals. The best motivators for fulfilling people's needs are the following:

- interesting and/or useful work
- a sense of achievement
- responsibility
- the opportunity for career progression or professional development
- gaining new skills and competencies
- a sense of belonging to one's work group/organisation.

Pride, lust, anger, gluttony, envy, sloth and covetousness are all listed as prime motivators, but hopefully not all of these are relevant to the medical environment to any great extent.

Developing a positive attitude

A positive outlook will combat many of the frustrations of everyday life at work and at home.

For a positive approach, use the following strategies.

- Concentrate on what you can do and not on what you cannot do.
- Accept your limitations – you are not superwoman/superman/super-housewife/superhusband/superspouse.
- Get things in perspective – don't become overwhelmed by demands; put problems and unhappy experiences behind you.
- Don't feel guilty about circumstances that are outside your control.
- Smile and actively think positive thoughts.
- Look for the humour in a situation whenever appropriate.
- Seek out and encourage other positive people; avoid continual whingers.
- Value yourself for being assertive.
- Take pride in your achievements.
- Think future commitments through and visualise yourself positively in control.
- Make positive plans to learn from mistakes.
- Communicate confidently.
- Use positive body language.

Being assertive

This may require you to learn assertiveness skills and practise them at every opportunity. Assertiveness is about knowing and practising your rights – to change your mind, make mistakes, not understand about something, refuse demands, express emotions and be yourself without having to act for other people's benefit.

Being assertive is about expressing your feelings clearly and openly and behaving in keeping with those feelings in an honest way. Being assertive is not the same as being aggressive. It is about deciding what you want to do or to happen, judging whether it is reasonable or not, and acting accordingly.

Assertiveness in the work context is about facing up to the fact that everyone has a limit to their time and energy, and politely but firmly refusing to take on extra work if you know that it will cause you to be overstretched. Refuse to be manipulated by others.

Assertiveness is certainly not about getting what you want all the time. It is about setting out your own boundaries, and being prepared to stick up for yourself if you think you are right, while at the same time being willing to reach a compromise with others. You should be able to learn skills to negotiate assertively with everyone – patients, senior and junior colleagues, and family members. It is about giving and taking in an equitable way.

You are not perfect at everything you do. You can use assertiveness to acknowledge your areas of weakness, and then plan to move forward with a particular activity or development.

To be successful in being assertive, you need to learn to recognise the tricks that others employ to get their own way. Some people can be devious, dropping hints about what they really want but placing the onus on you to decide exactly what it is. This is ridiculous. You have better things to do with your time and energy than play these kinds of games. Faced with these types of people, you need to state clearly and simply what you think is the best way forward and refuse to be sidetracked.

If people try to bully you, and persist even after you have told them 'no', don't give in. Giving in just for the sake of some peace and quiet will make things worse in the long run, and you will feel resentful as well as stressed. Keep saying calmly but firmly 'I don't think you heard me; I'm not prepared to do that.' It is important to resist the temptation to get angry. Disarm the anger of a patient, colleague or member of the family by acknowledging their feelings and staying calm – but do not give in.

Passive behaviour in others can be especially difficult to handle, as it is a technique health professionals may fall for if they feel selfish for ignoring the 'victim's' wishes or hesitant requests. Be careful. You might end up doing what the passive person wants you to do rather than living with the guilt of pleasing yourself. Respond by stating specifically what you want with a simple explanation. When the next person needles you by saying 'no one really cares any more about how people feel' or 'I expect it's all my fault' and you feel yourself tempted to reassure them to the contrary, think of the games that they are playing. They are trying to manipulate you. Don't fall for it!

One of the characteristics of someone who is healthily assertive is that they are not afraid to state their opinion. No one should be afraid to give their opinion on a subject they know something about. And not only do you have as much right to be heard as anyone else – you also have the right to change your mind. If you decide that on reflection you don't want to take on a task, don't be afraid to say so.

The potential advantages to you of being assertive are as follows:

- to increase your self-confidence
- to increase control over your emotions
- to establish better relationships with others – people will relate to assertive people more readily than to those who are passive or aggressive
- to increase your self-respect
- to increase respect from others
- to achieve satisfactory changes in your work or home situation.

Tips for assertiveness

1   Say '*No*' clearly and then move away or change the subject. Keep repeating '*No*' and don't be diverted.
2   Be honest and direct with everyone.
3   Do not apologise or justify yourself more than is reasonable.
4   Offer a workable compromise and negotiate an agreement that suits you and the other person.
5   Pause before answering a '*Yes*' that you will later regret. Delay your response and give yourself more time to think by asking for more information.
6   Be aware of your body language and keep it as assertive as possible. Match your tone to your words (don't smile if you are giving a serious message).
7   Use the 'broken-record' technique – persistently repeat your message in a calm manner to someone who is trying to pressurise you to do something that you do not want to do. Do not be side-tracked.
8   Show that you are listening to the other person's point of view and giving them a fair hearing.
9   Practise expressing your opinion and rights rather than expecting other people to guess what you want.
10   Don't be too hard on yourself if you make a mistake – everyone is human.
11   Be confident enough to change your mind if that is appropriate.
12   It can be assertive to say nothing at all.

Conclusion

These are just some of the skills that might be useful to you and the rest of your family. The particular skills that will help you are those that suit your own personality and style and the circumstances that you want to change.

Keep reflecting on which of the tools you are going to use as you continue reading through the book and make your logical plan (*see* Chapter 9).

References

1   Richards C (1989) *The Health of Doctors.* King's Fund, London.

2   Jones J, Hodgson J, Clegg T *et al.* (1998) *Self-Reported Work-Related Illness in 1995. Results from a household survey.* Health and Safety Executive, Sudbury.

3   Allen I, Hale R, Herzberg J *et al.* (1999) *Stress among Consultants in North Thames.* Policy Studies Institute, London.

4   Sibbald B and Young R (2001) *The General Practitioner Workforce 2000. Workload, job satisfaction, recruitment and retention.* National Primary Care Research and Development Centre, Manchester.

5   Evans J, Lambert T and Goldacre M (2002) *GP Recruitment and Retention: a qualitative analysis of doctors' comments about training for and working in general practice.* Occasional Paper 83. Royal College of General Practitioners, London.

6   Dumelow C, Littlejohns P and Griffiths S (2000) Relation between a career and family life for English hospital consultants: qualitative, semi-structured interview study. *BMJ.* **320**: 1437–40.

7   Scottish General Practitioners Committee (2001) *The Reality Behind the Rhetoric.* British Medical Association, Scottish Office, Edinburgh.

8   Caplan RP (1994) Stress, anxiety and depression in hospital consultants, general practitioners and senior health service managers. *BMJ.* **309**: 1261–3.

9   Chambers R and Campbell I (1996) Anxiety and depression in general practitioners: associations with type of practice, fundholding, gender and other personal characteristics. *Fam Pract.* **13**: 170–3.

10   British Medical Association (2002) *BMA Cohort Study of 1995 Medical Graduates. Seventh Report.* British Medical Association, London.

11   Cannon D (1996) *Generation X and the New Work Ethic.* Demos, London.

12   Huby G, Gerry M, McKinstry B *et al.* (2002) Morale among general practitioners: qualitative study exploring relations between partnership arrangements, personal style and workload. *BMJ.* **325**: 140–2.

13   Hart-Davis A (2002) Ten top tips for your happiness at work. *Evening Standard.* **30 August**: 17.

14   Maslow AH (1970) *Motivation and Personality.* Harper and Row, New York.

Further reading

- Chambers R (1999) *Survival Skills for GPs.* Radcliffe Medical Press, Oxford.
- Chambers R and Davies M (1999) *What Stress in Primary Care!* Royal College of General Practitioners, London.
- Chambers R, Hawksley B and Ramgopal T (1999) *Survival Skills for Nurses.* Radcliffe Medical Press, Oxford.
- Cox T (1993) *Stress Research and Stress Management: putting theory to work.* HSE Contract Research Report No. 61/1993. Health and Safety Executive, Sudbury.

5

Surviving time pressures

Time management is all to do with being smarter about getting through your work or your chores at home. A certain degree of time pressure is probably necessary for you to maintain your interest and momentum in getting a job done. However, too much pressure could tip you over the peak of your performance curve so that you are less efficient and your work or home life suffers as you become less effective.

Doctors are conditioned by their training and work to feel that they must cope, whatever the time pressures. They feel that patients must not suffer, whatever the costs to themselves. However, there are limits to your tolerance, and if too much pressure is exerted for too long a time, you may end up feeling burnt out and consequently have less energy for your family at home. Therefore you must learn to control the demands on your time, before any excessive pressures affect you and your performance adversely.

The key to good time management at work and at home is to:

- balance your work and leisure time
- prioritise how you spend your time – do not allow yourself or others to waste it
- control interruptions
- include time for thinking, doing, meeting and learning in your working day
- allow sufficient time for the unexpected
- delegate work whenever it is appropriate, both at work and at home
- try only to accept delegated work without further training if you have the necessary skills, time and experience to do so
- get on with essential tasks – do not procrastinate
- be assertive – learn to say 'no' often enough to unnecessary work or taking on other people's jobs and tasks
- make effective decisions – and don't look back
- put past mistakes behind you – do not ruminate over them
- review significant problems and learn to manage time better in order to avoid those problems in future by making realistic action plans.

In order to minimise the time pressures, you first need to identify the prime causes of such pressures as described in Chapter 4 and then make changes to reduce or avoid them as far as possible.

Control long working hours

When doctors constantly work the long hours reported by the GP in Box 5.1 below, they will become tired and demoralised, and their family life will suffer as a result.

Box 5.1:

I leave the house at 7a.m. and return at 7.30p.m. My children are teenagers now, but when they were small I never saw them during the week ... General practice is horrendously family-unfriendly.

(GP, aged 45)

At work you need to:

- optimise any time-saving arrangements to relieve you of tasks (e.g. by delegating work, recruiting more staff, becoming more expert at making the computer work for you)
- consider reducing your work commitment if you can afford to do so
- contemplate a move to a less pressured post or practice (e.g. where there is more help out of hours, or a higher doctor-to-patient ratio)
- if you stop doing a particular task or job, avoid letting the work that is left expand to fill your time
- see whether you can drop any commitments or sessional work that are external to the practice or department and which are not your core work
- develop a sensible policy (that everyone adheres to) for accepting extra and urgent patients on to surgery or clinic lists. Then you should be able to anticipate better what time your working day will end.

At home you need to:

- reassess the income that you need (can you live on less and drop some working hours?)
- review with your spouse or partner how you divide who does what with regard to outside work and home care (can you revise the hours you both work so that the balance is fairer for both of you?)
- delegate any domestic tasks that you can by employing help (in the house or garden) or childcare if that is what you need.

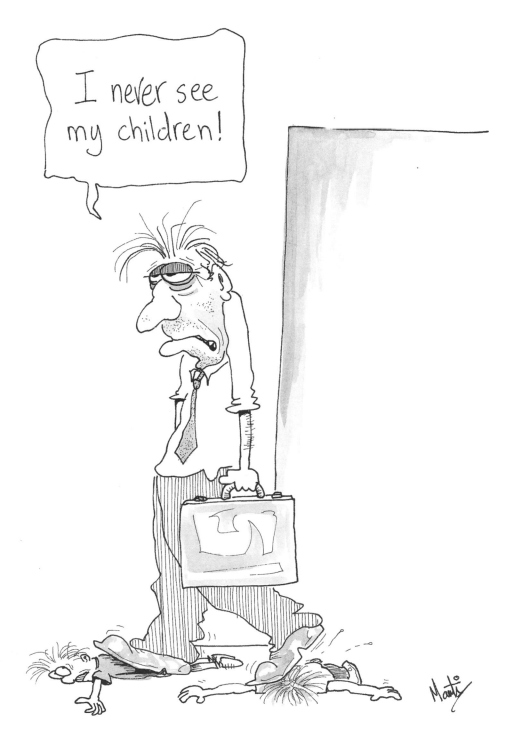

Limit interruptions

People are stressed by situations over which they have little control, such as interruptions. If you go into your department or practice early in order to catch up on paperwork, you will get little done and feel increasingly irritated if you receive incessant telephone calls or staff enquiries.

Interruptions are one of the biggest timewasters, especially if someone else could have handled the problem or taken the message, or if no action was required. Even if an interruption is necessary it may occur at the wrong time, wrecking your concentration or train of thought. Keep focused on your priorities and do not allow others to engage you in idle chat when you are intent on work or another activity.

At work you need to:

- restrict interruptions at designated times in order to clear your paperwork – ask staff to stall enquiries until you are available
- reorganise your systems at work to suit you better (but obviously you must be accessible sometimes)
- introduce a time when you are available for non-urgent requests.

At home you need to:

- agree times with your partner and children that are essential for you to be at home or at an activity outside work, and times when this is desirable. Plan your working day so that you stick to those essential times at least
- regard minutes or hours as *costed* time – think of how much some of the activities on which you spend time are worth, and whether different activities are of equal value.

Restrict paperwork

The excessive paperwork that seems to be an integral part of the health service is a potent cause of stress for all doctors, whatever the stage of their career. The Government runs exercises to cut the mounds of paperwork, but the demands of accountability seem to trigger escalating requirements for form-filling.

Many doctors do not have sufficient time to complete all of the essential paperwork during their working hours, and end up taking it home. There it looms over them, so that they do it in a half-hearted way when they are tired, thus ensuring that it takes even longer to finish.

At work you need to:

- never complete routine paperwork that can be delegated to support staff

- sign claim forms, etc., but do not fill in any other details – leave this to others
- carry a tape recorder with you and dictate requests for staff to complete tasks for you
- complete the most complicated paperwork first when you are still fresh
- never handle a letter or report more than once – read it and act on it. If you procrastinate you will waste time re-reading it later.

At home you need to:

- *never* bring routine paperwork home. Go in to work early the following morning and do it in half the time it would take at home, while you are still fresh.

Time yourself

You need to be more aware of how you spend your time. It is amazing how much unplanned time you can squander in social chat in the corridor or car park, or in discussion on the telephone.

At work you need to:

- review how well you keep to time on clinical work. If keeping to time is difficult and a major source of stress for you, consider altering the rate at which you book patients. If you always end 30 minutes late, consider booking longer time slots, but bear in mind the implications of this if you see the same number of patients over a longer time period
- organise your reference resources and records so that you can find information promptly without wasting time hunting for it.

At home you need to:

- keep a mental or written log of examples of situations where you are under time pressure. Think what you can do to avoid that pressure and change your habits accordingly (e.g. get up ten minutes earlier to walk the dog or to avoid the rush to work)
- review the time you take to do activities that you could avoid or delegate, and consider whether it is worth employing help (e.g. a gardener)
- limit the amount of time you spend on the telephone. If you measure how long you talk for the next few times you are on the phone, you will probably be surprised how long the calls last. Listen to yourself – you may find that much of the time is spent on pleasantries or repeating what you have already said.

Prioritise your time: do not allow yourself or others to waste it

Be clear about what your goals are for your work and home life, sport and leisure activities. The way in which you allocate your time will look very different if your main goal is to be a great golfer, or to learn a new skill such as aromatherapy or photography, or to spend as much time as possible with your family. Plan your goals in association with whoever else they affect, and make sure that if you have more than one goal they do not conflict.

Once you have clearly identified your goals, set out your strategies for achieving them. Then structure sufficient time around those priorities.

At work and at home you need to:

- log time spent on daily activities and map out the activities and tasks that are essential. Review the way in which you have spent your time compared with the goals and priorities that you have previously set out. If there is a discrepancy, think through the possible reasons for this and resolve on a new schedule
- match any new activity against your goals. If it takes you further away from your goals, then refuse to take it on, but if it brings you closer to achieving your goals, consider whether you have time to fit it in. Be firm with yourself and do not agree to do it just because you like the person who is asking you and want to please them
- spend your quality time doing the priority jobs. It is too easy to focus on getting small unimportant tasks done and put off tackling the large ones, which then just hang over you and make you feel guilty about leaving them unattended. Rate activities according to their priority – a high-priority task has to be done, a medium-priority task may be delegated or put off temporarily, and a low-priority task should only be done if you have no medium- or high-priority tasks waiting, or if you are feeling too jaded to tackle them
- concentrate on one task at a time. Complete it and then either move on to another job or take a short break to refresh yourself and clear your mind so that you are ready to start again. Do not move from one task to another or you will waste effort, as you will have to start thinking about the topic all over again each time you take it up.

Spend sufficient time reflecting, developing and learning

Time devoted to developing and learning is well spent and needs to be time-tabled in, not regarded as an activity to be fitted in only if there is sufficient slack time. You need to be fresh and creative in order to stay on top of the demands that are made on you as a doctor and remain productive. You can only manage this in the longer term if you have the right mix of stimulating work and personal and professional development within your daily schedule. Persistent overwork will be counter-productive and will also be a negative stress which may lead to your becoming less effective – and wasting time.

Allow time for the unexpected

Allow at least 10% of your time for dealing with unexpected tasks – both at work and at home. In the unlikely event that everything goes smoothly and you do not need the extra time, it will be a bonus to have that additional space in which to catch up on the backlog of paperwork, or simply to spend a little more time with your partner and family at home.

Be assertive: say 'no' to unnecessary work or other people's jobs and tasks

The greatest challenge is to be assertive with yourself so that you do not agree to take on additional tasks that are not essential for you to undertake, or that fall outside your own priority areas. If you are not careful you may become so busy helping others that you do not get your own work done (*see* Chapter 4 for ideas on being more assertive at work and at home).

Make effective decisions

Be decisive and finish the jobs in hand both at work and at home. Gather information about a problem or choice, weigh up the pros and cons with other people as appropriate, and then make a decision. Once you have made that decision, look forward and make plans for the future – do not look backward and frame regrets. Some tips on making effective decisions are listed below.

- There are always other options – find out what they are.
- Gather ideas and evidence from other people or from a range of sources – do not confine yourself to the options you already know about.
- Base your analyses and decisions on reliable objective evidence or observations, and not on 'guesstimates'. Effective decisions are based on reality, not on hope, so use probing questions to establish the facts.
- Think through the implications of your decisions by considering the possible consequences before choosing which options to take.

- Find out about feelings as well as facts – what the situation really is and how people feel about it.
- Your personality and beliefs will affect your decision making.
- Do not accept other people's perceptions of reality – look and think for yourself.
- Be honest with yourself and others, and maintain your integrity. The best decisions are based on truth, not on illusions.
- Simple decisions are usually the best ones, and are often obvious in retrospect.
- Fear gets in the way of making realistic assessments of the options.
- Do not make decisions because you are frightened of something, but because you are enthusiastic about the expected outcomes.

How you feel about the way in which you make a decision often predicts the results. If you feel good about a decision, the outcome is usually a success.

Make time for the family

On the whole, doctors tend to be caring people who give a lot of their attention and energy to their patients. This may leave them mentally, physically and emotionally drained, and conflict and resentment at home often result, unless the doctor's partner and children can adopt a mature and understanding attitude. It may seem to the child/children that their doctor–parent has time for everyone else except for their family, who should be most important in their list of priorities. It is not that no attention is being given to the child, but that it is perceived as being too little, which may result in the child seeking attention from other sources (not necessarily sensible ones).

Further reading

- Treacy D (1998) *Successful Time Management in a Week*. Hodder and Stoughton, London.

6

Listening and talking

At a recent social gathering, friends were discussing the old chestnut about how doctors seemed to be so poor at talking to patients, especially breaking bad news.

'If you ask me', said one, 'they train it out of them at medical school.'

However, the funny thing is, that those same people were quick to extol the virtues of their own GPs. This is not a new phenomenon. If you read the press, doctors in general are hopeless at talking to patients – they talk down to them, they keep them in the dark and they don't involve them in decision making – yet individual patients think that their own doctors do a great job.

Actually we think that one of the things we do well as doctors is both listen and talk to patients. Of course we don't always get it right, and the anxiety that hovers around consultations with patients can both get in the way of good communication and make recall of how it went difficult, but on the whole it is a large part of what we do. It would be surprising if, over time, we did not develop ways of understanding the things that patients are saying and talk to them in ways that make it easier for them to be involved.

One cause of dissatisfaction within busy households is poor communication. Earlier chapters have considered how this sometimes manifests itself and what we can do to build better relationships at home. This chapter starts by recognising that doctors already have the basics of good communication skills. Here we shall discuss how you can hone these skills for use at home, what happens when you don't listen, and how you can improve the way in which you talk to each other in your family.

> *He was but as the cuckoo is in June, heard not regarded.*
> (Shakespeare, Henry IV, 1: Act III, Scene ii)

How often has someone in your family told you that you are not listening to them (as Sam does about his doctor–father in Box 6.1)? Have you ever spent the evening talking to someone at home only to discover it was going 'in one ear and out the other'? Do your children ever preface any discussion with 'there's no point telling you, you wouldn't understand'? It is possible to increase the likelihood that if someone is speaking at home, someone is actually hearing what they are saying.

Box 6.1:

I know when Dad is not really listening. He tries to be interested, but he's really thinking about the last patient or how he can get the car serviced and still be able to do home visits. I know because he just sort of grunts and says 'uh-huh', and if I ask him a question he doesn't know what I'm talking about. And then he realises and he sort of looks at me hard and asks me again, but then there isn't any point.

(Sam, aged 11)

There are some general skills for good interpersonal communication, which are based on the technique of active listening.[1] First, it is important to listen with genuine interest. This means putting down what you are doing and paying attention to the person who is speaking. However, this also demands a degree of good timing on the part of the speaker. The children in our survey were very sophisticated about choosing the right moment to talk to their parents who were doctors (e.g. not when they first walked in through the door, or when they were busy at their desk with paperwork). However, having had their attention caught, the listener needs to show that the conversation matters and that they are taking in what is being said.

There is little point in trying to engage your son in a conversation about keeping his bedroom tidy when all of his friends are round to play football in the garden. By considering what effect our message will have on the listener and choosing the time and place when they are likely to be most receptive, we can show understanding and empathy for others, which is the second important point about good communication. Empathy means trying to see what it is about the story you are hearing that matters to the person who is telling you. Remember the perspective of the speaker. Comments such as 'it's only a game' do not help the 11-year-old who just failed to make the school team, any more than saying 'I never liked him' will help a teenage girl get over her first broken heart.

Be encouraging

It is not always possible to be positive when family members bring you sad or bad news to discuss. Perhaps your son has a disappointing school report, your husband did not get that important job, your wife has been overlooked for promotion or your mother has had a health scare. However, it is possible to be encouraging. Express your pride in their achievements, tell them what they mean to you, and look for other ways to increase their self-esteem and confidence. This does not mean being artificially upbeat when there is little to be celebrated, but it does mean looking for the positive aspects of situations and expressing challenges as opportunities.

Watch for minimal cues

Good interpersonal skills are built on an ability to respond to more than just the spoken word. Patients who are depressed often tell us that they are fine while looking at the floor and failing to make eye contact. We learn to look beyond the words to match the spoken and the non-spoken signals. This is sometimes called *non-verbal leakage* – that is, the discrepancy between what patients want to tell us and the messages that they are unconsciously transmitting. We can use the ability to detect this at home as well. Try not to ignore the 'it doesn't matter' throw-away comments made by someone who feels that you are preoccupied. You need to watch facial expressions, posture and muscle tension as well as the content, tone and speed of speech.

Sometimes it is not possible to get to the bottom of why a family member is upset, angry or anxious. Another skill from the consulting-room that might help is reflection. Repeat words or phrases that they have used and allow pauses for them to elaborate. In addition, skilful use of phrases such as 'so it seems to me that you are saying ...' enable you to summarise or paraphrase what you have heard in order to check understanding, demonstrate that you are listening and minimise opportunities for misunderstanding.

However, learning how to listen, or applying the listening techniques that you use at work to the conversations you have at home, is only half the battle. All good interpersonal communication depends on building a good relationship in the first place. Most busy families grow together over time and rarely stop to think about how those relationships are formed. And that is probably ideal. However, if things are not going well at home, either because of lack of time to spend together or because individual members are preoccupied with their own lives, then it might be worth stopping and working on the rapport within the family.

Building healthy relationships

It is important that the environment at home is conducive to a free exchange of information. Everyone should feel equally able to participate in family discussions and be included in family decision making. This means valuing all contributions, making a realistic attempt to explain things to younger members, considering all suggestions and being open to changing your mind. In any partnership there will be times when one member is more in need of support than the other. Each member of the family should feel equally able to assume the role of the one needing support as well as being a caregiver.

Adopt a similar language. Just as with patients, the language that we use can be a barrier to effective communication rather than an aid to it. As Oscar Wilde said of the English and the Americans, families can be 'divided by a common language'. All the time in the world spent talking as a family will not be helpful if some members feel excluded by the language because it is too technical, too involved or apparently not relevant to them, as the quote in Box 6.2 demonstrates.

Box 6.2:

I have always thought he brought his work home, I suppose we both do a bit. But now he brings home the way he speaks as well. He always says things three times because that's how he talks to patients. He says they forget what you say unless you drum it in. Well, I am not like that, once will do – if he explains it properly.

(Practice manager, wife of GP husband)

Some family members may complain of a lack of involvement in decision making. Sometimes this is entirely appropriate (deciding which bank to apply to for a mortgage is not a conversation you need to have with a 10-year-old), but sometimes you can be so used to making decisions and getting things done that you forget to involve others when their contribution would be useful. The use of plural pronouns to indicate partnership is a useful way of inviting contributions and demonstrating that you value all family members' thoughts. Phrases such as 'We could try ... what do you think?', 'Do you think it would help if we ...?' or 'Let's ask around and see what others have done' all invite involvement and sharing.

Not only do busy people make decisions without negotiation or involving others, but those in a household with someone who is apparently distracted by other outside responsibilities are also likely to get on with running things alone. This may work well, but however well meaning it is, it may lead to a sense of exclusion or result in others feeling that their opinions are not required.

It can also be helpful if decisions are phrased in provisional rather than dogmatic terms, whether or not there is joint discussion and ownership of that decision. So you could say to children 'Your mother and I think that ... but let's just give it a go and see what happens' rather than 'This is what we are doing – your mother and I have decided.' Any household with children will experience times when some behaviours are less than ideal. Potty training, toddler defiance, tantrums and expressions of individuality in teenagers are all areas of potential conflict, but also in a partnership there will be disagreements and irritations which, if left to fester, can become major sources of discontent. It is better to be 'up front' about behaviours that you find unhelpful, and all family members should feel that it is acceptable to raise such a subject. One way to make such discussions less likely to result in arguments is to phrase your comments in descriptive rather than judgemental terms. For example, 'Leaving soggy towels on the bathroom floor makes it harder for me to make sure there is a clean towel when you want a bath next' might be more effective than 'You are so lazy and untidy, the way you never hang the towels on the rail.' We stress the use of the word *might*. There is no accounting for some teenagers – but at least you tried, maintained your dignity and treated them with respect. They might just get the message (eventually) and learn from your example to treat others with respect.

In a similar vein, it is helpful to restrict comments that are likely to cause upset to the issues and not the person him- or herself, and to be specific in your criticisms. Sixteen-year-olds can get away with 'I hate you, you are ruining my life' because we know they are less articulate and are expressing pent-up anger and frustrations. This is less acceptable as we get older, and 'I really don't like the way you let me down when you said you could get the children from school and then changed your mind' is much more effective than 'You are so unreliable, you are always letting me down.'

It can be important to recognise and interpret your own feelings. If you are feeling uneasy and anxious, are others in the family feeling the same way, too? If you are angry, perhaps others are as well. Try just expressing how you feel. You might be surprised at the response from others.

So what if, having set aside time for family discussions, you cannot persuade family members to contribute? There is nothing worse than a partner or spouse who will not respond to your need to open a discussion. The underlying reasons will be important. Are they too tired, disinterested or angry? Is the timing wrong or have the reasons for the discussion not been made clear? Again you have skills that you can borrow from work to encourage participation.

Encourage the involvement of others

However you manage it, it is important to keep a dialogue going – it is difficult to share ideas with a monologue. As mentioned earlier, it is important to use shared language. Do not talk down to children – they respond remarkably well to being treated like adults and to a demonstration that their view is important. Just as patients find jargon and 'psychobabble' unhelpful, family members will see through an insincere attempt to 'hear what you're saying' and will be alienated by language that is taken straight from work.

Try to avoid one person dominating any discussions, and allow all family members to have a say. Encourage those who are less articulate or who are entrenched in a position to contribute and express how they are feeling. Raised voices are not helpful, nor are long lectures. Urge everyone to explain their position and do not allow assumptions to go unchallenged.

Just as with patients, open questions can be used for exploration. Such questions encourage others to describe their position and cannot be answered with a simple 'yes' or 'no'. They are a good way to define others' beliefs and feelings. For example, 'Tell me about your day' is more helpful than 'have you had a good day?'. Closed questions on the other hand are useful for obtaining facts and clarification. They are helpful if a conversation has completely stalled, but they should be used with caution. For example, they may reinforce a teenager's belief that you have no understanding of their world if you show that you are not on their wavelength by your closed questioning. The conversation in Box 6.3 has been repeated in one form or another at many a school gate.

Box 6.3:

'Have you had a nice day?'
'Not bad.'
'Why were you so late coming out? I've been here ten minutes.'
'Don't know.'
'Is it that boy in Year 6 again?'
'No.'
'So everything's OK?'
'Yes.'
'Good. What do you want for tea?'

If a situation at home has become very tense due to ineffective communication and misunderstandings coupled with inconsiderate behaviour over a prolonged period, giving others the opportunity to express how they feel may seem quite threatening. Being respectful of each other's feelings, giving encouragement, maintaining eye contact and being interested in each other will be a good start. It may be necessary to agree some ground rules for group discussions if that is a setting which your family is not used to or with which it does not feel comfortable. Such rules might include not interrupting each other, avoiding the use of personal remarks and offensive language, and a common agreement about the purpose of the meeting.

Having grasped the nettle of opening a discussion about relationships at home, or difficult decisions that need to be made, how can you encourage change in yourself or others? Planning for change takes all of the skills of effective communication we have outlined already, as well as a true ability to see things from another's perspective. We need to understand the impact that any changes will have on another person, and anticipate what their reactions are likely to be.

Planning changes

Try to make it easy for the person concerned to change or fit in with the changes that need to be made. For example, if you want children to keep their bedrooms tidy, make sure that there is enough storage space. People are more likely to follow plans if they are not overwhelmed with tasks to do, if the plan fits with the way in which they look at things or with other tasks that they have to do, and if they have the necessary capacity and resources. For example, children can be encouraged to help around the house if they are given interesting manageable tasks that they can develop and take a pride in. Success is less likely if they are bored, feel that there is too much to do or are always being nagged at.

Think of the context within which the changes need to be made. Can other family members help? Does it have to be Mum who takes the dog for a walk or could there be a rota that fits in with other family activities?

Given that it may not always be necessary, desirable or possible to involve everyone in the family in decision making, it will still be necessary to take their perceptions into account. Change is more likely to be implemented if the actions and outcomes seem to be important to everyone, if they understand why change is important and if they believe that the change is necessary.

Finally, like every other difficult aspect of family life, it all becomes much easier if there is mutual respect.

Conclusion

Some of these skills need time and practice before they can be used with confidence and without seeming too artificial. To complete the analogy with skills used in the consultation, you can use a checklist modified from one developed for analysing effective consultations in order to assess your effectiveness with relationships at home.[1] Try asking yourself the questions listed in Box 6.4 after any difficult conversation with a family member.

> **Box 6.4:**
>
> Do I know significantly more about the other person's perspective than before we started?
> Was I curious?
> Did I listen?
> Did I find out what mattered to them?
> Did we get to the nub of the issue?
> Did we share options in the discussion?
> Did we share the decision making?
> Did we check with each other to see if we really understood each other?
> Did we agree?

Reference

1   Tate P (2003) *The Doctor's Communication Handbook* (4e). Radcliffe Medical Press, Oxford.

7

Making the most of time off duty with your partner and family

Spouses or partners will eventually feel neglected if the doctor is completely wrapped up in his or her work, and their relationship is gradually weakened. No family is immune from the pressures of modern life, and doctors' families may suffer if the doctor–parent is worn down by caring for others. You will gain some insight into the way doctors' families feel from reading the report in Box 7.1 by a teenager from a family in which both parents are doctors.

Box 7.1:

No doubt all working parents find stress within their working environment, and will pass it on to their families through some form. However, due to doctors working an incredible amount of hours under a lot of stress, they ultimately find it harder to switch off, as they seem to be subconsciously thinking about the day's work and what tomorrow has in store for them.

It is not the job that affects a doctor's family, but the responsibilities that are brought with it. Doctors' children have probably experienced their parent(s) being disengaged from family life because of workload, and other such stresses, which they are forced to cope with every day at work. It is forgotten that they have to deal with the emotional aspects of being a doctor, as they deal with a wide variety of patients who all have different problems in their lives which may not only be medical. These issues need to be addressed with the same attention as their medical problems, where doctors still have to treat patients to the best of their ability. Children don't look at the stresses and pressures that their parent is inevitably being faced with, but concentrate on what they think is lacking in family life due to their parent's dedication to work.

(Hifsa, aged 17)

Balance your work and leisure time successfully

One of the ways to reduce stress both at work and at home is to timetable enough free time during your day to give you space for rest and relaxation to counteract the stresses and strains.

Try to complete work activities within your normal working hours, so that you have enough time for non-work-related activities in your life. If you do not allow sufficient time for leisure you will not have the opportunity for personal growth outside work and will probably become stale. Every so often you might set a target to learn or improve at something outside work, or take active measures to nurture your relationship with your spouse or partner, family and friends (e.g. by sharing a new hobby).

Make regular time and space for yourself for fun, relaxation, hobbies and enjoying simple pleasures throughout your life as a *stress-proofing* measure. Do not suddenly try to adopt these methods to beat stress at one particular time in your working life, when you are already below par. One of the best ways to monitor whether you are managing to protect enough time for yourself is to keep a daily log of activities for a week or so. At a recent clinical update meeting the lecturer asked the medical audience to be honest and indicate how much time they had spent in the previous week pursuing an activity that was for *their own* enjoyment. Only a quarter of the audience could say that they had done this – a sad state of affairs.

Sort your daily activities into three separate columns:

- *personal needs*, including shopping, sleeping, domestic chores, bodily needs, etc.
- *work*, including reading work-related books, reports and papers
- *leisure*, including sport, relaxation, reading, music, etc.

Work out the totals for the types of activities for each day. Then compare your daily recordings with the national recommendations for a healthy lifestyle by grouping your activities into the following categories:

- 45–55% on personal needs
- 25–30% on work
- 20–25% on leisure.

When your work component increases above 25%, it is the leisure proportion of your day that is usually reduced.

Family priorities

Regularly re-evaluate those extra commitments that are keeping you away from your family, especially if these are in the evening, at night or at weekends, and see if there are any which you might drop or change (as the medical politician in Box 7.2 did).

Box 7.2:

A prominent medical politician astounded his medicopolitical colleagues by resigning from national committees such as the BMA Council, the General Practitioners Committee and the Local Medical Committee after many years in these roles. He explained that the political work had kept him away from his family, and that his two teenage children were growing to resent the time he spent away from them.

Get work-related worries off your chest when you come home, and then put them aside. Consider delegating some of the activities which need to be done if you are running a home, working and raising a family. Perhaps employ a cleaner or a gardener, get some help with ironing or decorating, and/or collaborate with other parents to share the ferrying of children to school and different activities.

Try to prioritise time for events that are important to your children or partner. Consider the anguish it causes if the doctor is not present for key fixtures in their child's school or sporting life (*see* Box 7.3).

Box 7.3:

There are negative aspects to the job (of a doctor), but these are normally due to the effects on the rest of the family as a result of the lifestyle that they are forced to live. A doctor's inflexible work hours mean that they miss events that are important to their child. Even though the child knows this is unavoidable, they will inevitably feel resentful and upset at their parent for missing events such as Sports Day at school, where they were one of the only ones whose Mum/Dad didn't compete in the Mums' and Dads' races, or a swimming gala where they won the gold medal in the 50 m front crawl by half a stroke. They want to share the occasion with both parents, but more importantly they want their parents to feel proud. Even being told later in the evening isn't the same, as discussing the event later isn't the same as witnessing it there.

(Doug, aged 13)

Whole family approach

Doctors' families often have to overcome the fact that one parent has to take on the main caring role. This can create a stressful environment at home, as that parent struggles to balance the housework with the shopping and picking the kids up from school, etc. Instead of a calm environment for the doctor to come home to which helps him or her to unwind, there is added tension which is sensed by the other members of the family. The doctor–parent who is working long hours can often feel that they are bonding less with their offspring due to their prolonged absence, and this may cause problems with their relationships with the rest of the family.

Many of the doctors' children to whom we spoke thought that the family should all put allocated time aside at least once a week, where the family get together to do something. This may be difficult, especially with older children who lead separate social lives and do not want to be embarrassed by being seen out with their parents. Such meetings might involve sitting round the table for a meal and discussing things that everyone is finding stressful at work and at school, or a new activity that everyone can join in, as Michael describes in Box 7.4.

Box 7.4:

Michael told us how his family had enrolled in an arts and crafts workshop that was run one evening a week at a nearby college. Despite having to miss a few of the sessions due to his father having to do extra work at his general practice, Michael was finding it easier to communicate with both parents, but especially with his father. He advised other doctors' families to find a mutual interest and take it up in the same way that his family had. He had had a pessimistic view about doing the activity together before he started, but in fact it seemed to have been very successful in bringing everyone together and allowing them to have fun.

Several doctors' children told us that 'family meetings' were a good idea. A different person in the family can think up a discussion topic each week, and time is taken to sit and discuss or even debate different outlooks on the given subject. However, the young people who suggested this approach recommended that the gathering should not be round a table, but in a more relaxed environment (e.g. in the lounge or out for a meal).

If you try to bring the family together more, you will have to be careful that the discussions do not alienate the children further. The example of Tim in Box 7.5 highlights our earlier warning in Chapter 6 that the language you use with the family at home should be pitched at everyone's level and interest.

Box 7.5:

Tim is 13 years old. He lives with his mother, father and younger sister. Both of his parents are doctors, but he doesn't really have many problems with that. However, he does admit that he has never experienced anything else so he doesn't really know how it is affecting him in comparison with others of his age. The thing that he objects to strongly is the discussions that the family has over dinner. He feels excluded, as he doesn't understand the medical lingo that is frequently used between his parents, and he rarely understands the topic of conversation as it is related to work. Tim thinks that his parents are too involved with work and he sometimes wishes that they would forget about work, at least while they are at home.

Tim's younger sister demands a lot of attention, and he finds that because his parents are so busy it is normally his responsibility to keep her occupied. This annoys him, as in the evenings his time needs to be dedicated to schoolwork and she distracts him. Furthermore, at weekends his friends come round and his sister demands attention then as well. She is a complete pain and he wishes that his parents would tell her to leave him alone, but instead they tell him not to pick on her. Tim says this is because they welcome the break from her to do their own work and they don't care that she annoys him.

Enjoying your children

Try to arrange times when your children have your full attention. Talk about your work with them so that they can be more understanding about your being away from home. Try to take more interest in what the children are up to and give them more praise when you can. That means overcoming any tendency you might have to praise only academic or sporting success.

The time you organise with your children should be quality time, not just those occasions when you are too fatigued to do anything else (*see* Box 7.6). Doctors' children, even at a very young age, realise that if one or both of their parents work long hours they may seem to be withdrawn from family life. To a certain extent they accept this as just one of those things. It is only later in life when they are able to look back more critically on their earlier childhood that they start to see how their lives have been affected by their parent's chosen career, especially when they compare themselves with friends who live a different lifestyle due to their parents' more relaxed work patterns.

Box 7.6:

Mum never feels like playing games because she has so much work to do, but when she does join in you can tell that she doesn't really want to, and she always asks how long it will be until we can finish.

(Ann, aged 11)

Rebuilding your personal relationship with your spouse or partner at home

Various research studies of doctors in the UK and the USA have shown differences between male and female doctors' lifestyles. Fewer female than male doctors are married, female doctors have a higher divorce rate, and fewer female doctors than male have children.[1,2] Other research in the USA has shown that doctors are significantly more likely to have 'poor' marriages compared with non-medical couples (in that study 'poor' was defined as the marriage being 'unstable', or the sexual relationship being 'not as good as wished', or divorce having been casually considered).[3] Other researchers from the UK have described the strain on a marital relationship that is caused by a doctor's work.[4–6] Lack of time together, poor communication, lack of intimacy, intense preoccupation with work, the partner's resentment of the doctor's work, and frequent house moves all contribute to marital disharmony.

So another approach is to try to inject some freshness into your relationship with your partner, to strengthen the bond. Make a date as in the old days, and try to arrange regular outings for shared activities or interests. Acknowledge any problems with your sex life if they exist. These are usually due to communication difficulties or lack of time alone together. If you make rebuilding your relationship a priority and show a little patience, you will probably find some fun and laughter bubbling to the surface.

It is important to understand how your being a doctor may affect your relationship with your partner and the rest of the family. Your partner may feel increasingly resentful if they think that you are neglecting them as a result of your preoccupation with work. Your partner may be shouldering most of the responsibility for child rearing.[7] If you come home tired and irritable and your partner has been waiting for you, they will be disappointed and perhaps angry if you are detached and offhand towards them.

Therefore you need to spend time negotiating roles between you and your partner. Arrange the maximum dependable help to relieve the parent who has most domestic responsibilities where appropriate.

Keep working at establishing good and continuing communication in your marriage or long-term relationship. A counsellor from Relate might be helpful if your relationship is under threat, and you should seek such help sooner rather than later. Doctors have a tendency to delay seeking help.

The following ten suggestions for people who are married to a junior hospital doctor can be generalised to most medical marriages or long-term relationships.[8]

1 Get to know your partner well before you get married, so that you both know what you are letting yourselves in for.
2 Get married quite late to give you both plenty of time to get used to having your own lives.
3 Treat time together as precious and to be used in enjoying each other's company, not as an opportunity to moan about the bits you don't like.
4 Don't always expect to come first.
5 Don't ever keep meals waiting until your partner gets home. Eat when you need to and then get on with your life.
6 Make up your minds well in advance whose career comes first. If you are the one whose job is deemed to be more movable, be prepared to move cheerfully when the time comes.
7 If you are married to a hospital doctor, don't bother to spend weekends with him or her in hospital – the surroundings are awful.
8 Remember that life wasn't meant to be easy. No one forced you to marry a junior hospital doctor. Don't spoil it by concentrating on the bad bits.
9 If you really don't like it ... get a divorce and marry a teacher instead if you want to spend undisturbed nights, weekends and 12 weeks' holiday a year with someone else.
10 Love, determination, honesty and hope are all necessary, but you will have a lot more fun if you add laughter, optimism, cheerfulness and a positive approach to life as well.

Take time out

Plan and take regular holidays. If you and your medical colleagues have domestic responsibilities which mean that holidays can only be taken at specific times, negotiate your leave at the beginning of each year so that everyone knows what time they are taking and when. The improved quality of life may justify the time spent organising this – ask the family!

However, remember that a holiday does mean just that. However busy you are, there is no excuse for sneaking your work into your hand luggage thinking that you will catch up when the family is otherwise engaged (*see* Box 7.7).

Box 7.7:

Spare time is a good thing within a doctor's family. There are lots of exotic destinations to visit with accommodation of higher class than for a lot of families, because doctors have a good income. However, even though evenings and holidays are put aside for family time, they can be dominated by paperwork. I'm sure I am not the only doctor's daughter who has had to share my aeroplane seat with a laptop and various other files that I have moved when trying to secure some more legroom.

The holiday always seems slightly incomplete because of the workload that has to be taken with us. Even though the rest of us manage to enjoy ourselves in the pool and on the beach, the picture of Mum lying on a lounger in her swimming costume with the suntan lotion in one hand and work in the other seems somewhat wrong. Even when it comes to taking photographs, we have to throw a towel over the stack of paperwork and any other clue that work had to be taken with us, just in case anyone looks at our holiday snaps and questions it. Despite being miles away from the workplace, stress is still prominent, leading to perhaps more family arguments than are necessary on what should be a relaxing family holiday, but more importantly a care-free holiday.

(Viv, aged 15)

Make time for sport and hobbies – both to keep fit and to have fun.

Invest time in maintaining your network of friends

If you are preoccupied by work, your network of friends will gradually wither away if you do not have time for joint activities or to repay hospitality. Doctors' frequent moves around the country during the early stages of their careers make it more difficult to maintain friendships.

So timetable your friends into your busy lives when you are reviewing how you manage your time (*see* Chapter 5). Your children will probably enjoy time spent with other families, too (*see* Box 7.8).

Box 7.8:

My Dad has loads of friends through being a doctor, and we get to go out with them often for meals or to their houses. Lots of them have children that are my age, too, so I have made loads of new friends because of it.

(Prasad, aged 11)

References

1   Ducker DG (1986) *Health Thyself.* Brunner/Mazel, New York.

2   Allen I (1992) *Part-Time Working in General Practice.* Policy Studies Institute, London.

3   Vaillant G, Sobowale N and McArthur C (1972) Some psychological vulnerabilities of physicians. *NEJM.* **287**: 372–5.

4   Pereira Gray J (1982) The doctor's family: some problems and solutions. *J R Coll Gen Pract.* **32**: 75–9.

5   Hall A (1988) Medical marriage: no bed of roses. *BMJ.* **296**: 152–3.

6   Ward S (1994) GP spouses take the strain. *BMA News Rev.* **August**: 24–5.

7   Chambers R and Campbell I (1996) Gender differences in general practitioners at work. *Br J Gen Pract.* **46**: 291–3.

8   Montgomerie L (1992) Ten suggestions for getting the best out of (a hospital doctor's) life. *BMJ.* **305**: 120.

8

What happens when a doctor or a member of their family is ill?

If a doctor is ill and remains at work, their ill health may mean that the quality of patient care they provide is below par.

When a doctor is ill

Doctors often treat themselves when they are ill. Most doctors don't like being patients, and try to look after themselves (*see* Box 8.1). They order their own investigations, use medication that has been discarded by their patients or provided as free samples by pharmaceutical reps, and they refer themselves to consultant specialists.[1]

Box 8.1:

Dad is often feeling ill, but being a doctor he refuses to take medical advice and diagnoses himself. He says all he needs is a good night's peace without my younger brothers and sisters arguing. I think he is too stressed at work and needs to address some ways to reduce the stress, and I think that will make things a lot better at home.

(Sue, aged 17)

Doctors' children are very aware of their parents' struggles, as Dan's insight about his father's unhealthy lifestyle reveals in Box 8.2.

Box 8.2:

I know when my Dad is finding it hard at work because he smokes more when he's at home, and also he watches a lot more TV.

(Dan, aged 13)

Various surveys have reported the extent of self-treatment among doctors. In Staffordshire, nine out of ten doctors who had taken antibiotics had 'prescribed' these for themselves and, more worryingly, half of those taking antidepressant drugs had self-medicated.[1] A third of those having blood tests had initiated the test themselves, and a fifth of those having a chest X-ray had ordered the investigation for themselves.

Some doctors even go as far as performing surgery on themselves, as did one who reportedly performed his own vasectomy with the aid of his wife (*see* Box 8.3).

Box 8.3:   Doctor who performed a 'do-it-yourself' vasectomy

A good example of a doctor treating himself that hit the headlines in the medical press and national newspapers was that of a GP in West Sussex performing his own vasectomy in his own surgery, assisted by his wife (who is his practice manager) along with his practice nurse.

Dr H was reported as saying that the procedure hardly hurt, and that within a couple of days he was cycling to visit his patients at home. He justified performing the operation on himself by explaining that he knew of no other doctor who was competent to undertake a vasectomy who was as kind and careful as himself. As an experienced operator, he had performed 300–400 vasectomies. The GP had not forewarned the practice nurse, who was shocked when he called his wife in to assist and then performed his own operation after completing vasectomies on three other patients.

Newspaper reporters quizzed the General Medical Council (GMC) about their role or responsibility when doctors undertake surgery on themselves. The GMC responded that they are only able to remind doctors that they should avoid treating themselves or close family members. There is no action that they are required to take in such circumstances.

Doctors find it difficult to adopt the role of the patient for various reasons. Sometimes it is because they feel that they do not have enough time to go and see another doctor or health professional, to make an appointment to consult a doctor or return for follow-up care.

At other times, doctors may be embarrassed to admit that they are ill, as they regard their symptoms as a sign of weakness which they prefer to keep secret and cope with themselves. One research study in Northern Ireland found that GPs felt under pressure to appear physically well, and thought that patients believed a doctor's health reflected his or her own competence as a doctor.[2] Doctors were quoted as having said 'nobody wants to see a doctor who is sick' and 'unless you're unable to get out of bed you'll crawl in and work'.

Sadly, this attitude is sometimes perpetuated by colleagues who should be in a position to guide junior doctors towards a more positive approach to looking after their own health. The story of Tim in Box 8.4 illustrates this.

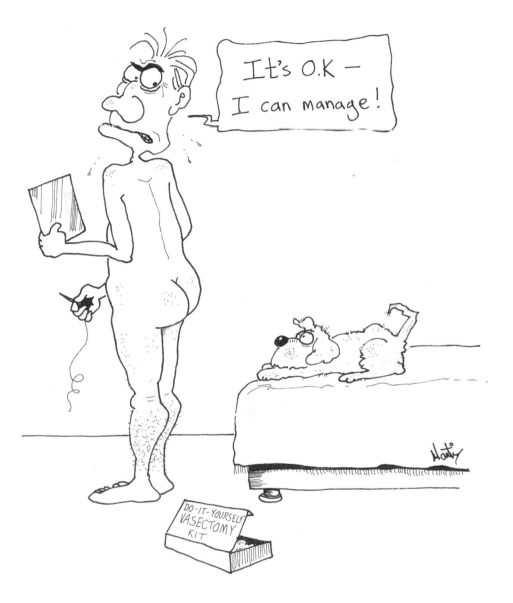

Box 8.4:

Alan, a senior and well-respected GP, took little heed when Tim, his GP registrar, became ill while on duty. Tim recalls 'I was on call all weekend with a horrible chest infection, and come Sunday night was coughing up blood. I phoned my trainer [Alan] and said I might not make it into surgery on the Monday. He said that everyone gets colds and how would it be if we all started acting like the patients?'.

Privacy can sometimes be a problem. A sick doctor may be self-conscious about being treated at a hospital as a patient. As one doctor said, 'you don't want to go and see your local psychiatrist in case one of your patients is sitting beside you in the waiting-room'.

It can be particularly difficult for a doctor to consult a medical colleague with whom they have a close working or social relationship, and to disclose personal matters. A considerable number of GPs are registered with doctors in their own practices instead of with GPs with whom they do not have a close working or personal relationship. If a doctor treats a work colleague, either or both of them might be embarrassed by the doctor taking a full history or performing a physical or mental examination. For the female GP described in Box 8.5 the embarrassment was caused by a personal examination by a midwife who was usually a work colleague.

Box 8.5:   Doctor too embarrassed to accept treatment by midwife colleague

One female GP who was registered with her own practice was reluctant to let the local midwife, whom she knew as a colleague, take out the stitches from her episiotomy when non-disposable sutures were used. She persuaded her husband to remove them with his Stanley knife (using a new blade!) the evening before her midwife colleague was due to visit.

Close colleagues may be prejudiced about possible differential diagnoses, or may allow their feelings to interfere with their professional objectivity. They may collude if the doctor denies that they have a health problem, especially if there is any threat to their livelihood. Colleagues may let their own interests override those of the doctor–patient (e.g. by pressurising them to return to work after their illness to help shoulder the workload of the practice, as described in Box 8.6).

Sometimes the sick doctor has such low self-esteem that they do not want to trouble another busy doctor, or even risk being mocked for over-inflating the importance of their signs and symptoms, so they do not seek medical help when they should do so.

Box 8.6:

Ron suffers from Crohn's disease and has had periodic flare-ups over the years. During one exacerbation he underwent a bowel resection and ileostomy. He was registered with Mike, one of the other GPs in his own practice. When the time came for reviewing his sickness certificate at two months, Ron faced overwhelming pressure to return to work as soon as possible, even though he was still feeling somewhat debilitated. He had taken out his sickness insurance policy *after* developing Crohn's disease, so was not covered by the policy. This meant that after the initial four weeks of sickness absence, when the practice paid for a locum, Ron had had to cover the locum's costs. When Ron consulted Mike two months after his major operation, his tentative suggestion that he return to work was immediately endorsed by Mike, as Mike's own workload had increased as a result of Ron's absence, and Mike's wife was complaining about this at home.

Doctors have a tremendous sense of duty about going to work and not letting their medical colleagues and patients down by taking sick leave. As one group of GPs said, 'You don't stay off work because you are not going to earn money. You continue to work because of your GP partners.'[2] This sense of duty is illustrated by the story of Pete in Box 8.7.

Box 8.7:

My mother is suffering from severe stress but won't take the day off work. She keeps telling me about how much money is lost each year because of people who don't turn up for work. She says if she was to take the day off then it would only mean more work for everyone else and for her, too, when she went into work the next day.

(Pete, aged 16)

One study found that the reasons given by consultants and GPs for 'working through' illness included awareness that absence would lead to an increased workload for colleagues, problems with adopting a patient role, and organisational barriers to taking sickness absence[3] (*see* Box 8.8).

Box 8.8:

My Dad often feels ill because of all the stress he's under at work. He says he can't take the day off because of all the stress it will cause other doctors with having to deal with his patients, and it will add to their workload. He never feels 100% well and is always tired.

(Liz, aged 15)

So the sick doctor may well deny their poor health and make light of their symptoms, even to the extent that their family life breaks down (*see* Box 8.9). Sometimes they deny their physical symptoms, and finally present with serious illnesses, such as cancer, late in the course of the disease.

Box 8.9:

My Mum and Dad got divorced last year because of the tension in the house. I think that it is mainly to do with the amount of stress my Mum was under. She became depressed and got angry really easily, but that could be because she frequently had difficulty sleeping. It put a strain on the whole family and we didn't know if we could do anything to help. She is now considering working part-time because the pressures at work are still there. I hope she does.

(John, aged 14)

There are plenty of reports in the medical press of comments made by the colleagues of doctors who have committed suicide, who realised too late that the doctor had been under severe stress (*see* Box 8.10). Suicide rates among male and female doctors are several times higher than those in the general population and in other professional groups.[4]

Box 8.10:   Some comments made by colleagues after doctors' suicides

Dr T seemed 'bomb-proof', but privately he was in very great difficulty and was struggling. This is almost the opposite of his public persona.

Dr G was so busy looking after his commitments and patients that he didn't have time to look after himself.

Dr M was one of those very conscientious and caring doctors who tend to take things to heart. Had her workload not been so great she would have coped admirably.

General practice does not suit everyone – you have to be thick-skinned and she was not. The pressure is such that you can't do the job properly, and she found that very difficult to cope with. She ended up with all the heartsink patients and she found it very difficult to say 'no' to people.

One common health problem among doctors is the misuse of alcohol and drugs. As many as 7% of doctors may suffer from some form of dependence on alcohol or drugs in their lifetime.[5] Doctors from all branches of medicine are affected. There are several confidential services to help addicted doctors (e.g. the Sick Doctors' Trust; tel. 01252 345 163). The partner and children of a doctor who is addicted to alcohol or drugs will suffer, too.

These days, everyone fears that confidential information about their ill health might inadvertently be leaked beyond those who need to know it. When a doctor is ill this can be a news story that is gossiped about among staff and patients. Examples of such breaches of confidentiality occur when correspondence from the hospital is opened by a secretary, or nosy staff rifle through medical notes without authority, or the doctor's casenotes feature in an external audit without being sufficiently anonymised.

Some solutions
Avoid self-diagnosis and self-treatment

It cannot be emphasised strongly enough that when doctors need medical advice for health problems they should not treat themselves or their work colleagues except with over-the-counter medication as any member of the public would do. It is tempting to cut corners, gain a quick opinion or take medication that is to hand. However, the self-treated or half-treated doctor–patient will be unlikely to receive good medical management unless they consult another doctor or health professional who works independently of them, and whose opinion they trust. The British Medical Association's guidelines on ethical responsibilities with regard to treating doctor–patients provide a good summary.[6]

- It is not advisable for doctors to assume responsibility for diagnosis and management of their own health problems, or those of their immediate family.
- All doctors should be registered with a GP, and hospitals should ensure that all staff have access to primary care and give staff time to attend a surgery where appropriate.
- Responsibility for overall care and continuity of treatment for doctors and their families should rest with their GP. Referral for a consultant's advice should go through the GP.
- It is preferable that the doctor's GP should not be a relative or, if feasible, a partner (at work).
- It is not advisable for doctors to prescribe themselves anything other than over-the-counter medicines.
- Doctors need to be aware that they become the patient in the doctor–patient partnership when receiving medical care.
- Doctors have an ethical duty to ensure that their own problems are effectively managed.
- Doctors should not take advantage of the access they have to medical records to look at the records of their family and friends.
- Doctors have a responsibility to ensure that they are protected against infectious diseases such as tuberculosis and hepatitis B.

- Doctors should not undermine the confidence that their relatives have in their own GP by being disparaging about the advice and treatment that they receive.

Be clear what practical help you need in order to remain at or return to work

You would think that health professionals and managers would realise what proactive help doctors and other colleagues need in order to be able to continue working if they are disabled by ill health of some kind. However, this is not usually the case, especially if the disabled or sick doctor conceals their impairment and is reluctant to ask for specific help or allowances to be made for their disability.

Team members who are under pressure from the heavy workload may feel resentful of a colleague whom they perceive as not pulling their weight because of their disability. Examples might include difficulty in visiting patients at home because of their poor sight or immobility, or periods of sickness absence for relapses of a chronic condition.

A doctor who develops a disability in mid-career will need to adapt their day-to-day life and environment. This will mean the rest of the team arranging working hours in as flexible a way as possible to suit both the person with the disability and the needs of the rest of the team. A doctor who is becoming progressively disabled by multiple sclerosis will be able to remain at work for longer if the practice premises are adapted externally and internally – in line with the Disability Discrimination Act – so that everywhere is accessible to someone sitting in a wheelchair or walking with elbow crutches. A disabled car parking space near the doctor's entrance to the surgery will help with access. Practice systems should be reorganised to allow the disabled doctor to consult on equal terms with able-bodied colleagues. A doctor or other member of staff with deteriorating vision will require improved lighting in office and surgery consulting-rooms, with complex magnifying aids and other vision equipment to hand. As their disability worsens, the doctor will need to be able to negotiate flexible working hours or conditions and reduce their work commitment, perhaps doing proportionally more office-based work and less domiciliary or other external work.

Look out for doctor colleagues

You need to make a special effort to look out for any colleagues who are not coping as well as usual, but who are keeping up the pretence that all is well.

Life events such as bereavement, marriage, divorce, childbirth and moving house are all major causes of stress. Such stresses are cumulative and spill over to affect work. It may be that the person is more irritable than they used to be, criticising and picking fault so that they alienate the very colleagues and friends whose support they most need. So look below the surface if a colleague seems to be behaving differently from usual, especially if they have had any significant life events in the recent past. Even if there is no apparent reason for their change in behaviour, keep probing gently, as they may be concealing a complaint lodged against them, an alcohol-related problem or some other source of distress.

The rehabilitation of colleagues who have been off work for several months will be made easier if they can start back part-time and phase in their return to work. They will probably lack confidence in their medical knowledge and skills and need support and encouragement from others.

Early retirement

Occasionally doctors retire early on health grounds, due to either mental health problems or physical disability which they attribute to their medical work. However, doctors are less likely to take early retirement on health grounds than some other health professionals (*see* Box 8.11).

Box 8.11: Retirement due to ill health in the NHS workforce

The relative rates of retirement on ill-health grounds reflect how well the various disciplines within the NHS workforce are faring at work. The overall rate of retirement due to ill health in the NHS was 5.5 per 1000 employees in England and Wales in 1998–99.[7]

Ambulance workers had the highest rates of ill-health retirement, with 15 out of 1000 retiring in 1998–99, compared with nurses (5 out of 1000), doctors (5 out of 1000) and healthcare assistants or support staff (13 out of 1000).[7] Two-thirds of the ambulance workers and half of the nurses retired because of musculoskeletal disease problems, compared with a quarter of the doctors. One-third of the doctors, one-fifth of the nurses, one-tenth of the healthcare assistants or support staff and one-sixth of the ambulance workers who retired on the grounds of ill health in the year reported did so for psychiatric reasons.

Reduce factors that cause ill health

As mental ill health in doctors is associated with an excessive workload, it makes sense to reduce and control that workload. Depression has been shown to be associated with having little free time from medical work, working on call, exhaustion and stress.[8,9]

Therefore doctors should review their life–work balance and ensure that they have enough time spent off duty to enable them to relax, keep fit and *enjoy* themselves (*see* Chapter 5 on time management for ideas on controlling any urge you have to work all hours).

When a member of the doctor's family is ill

When the doctor's child is ill

Gender inequality with regard to roles and responsibilities for childcare and domestic tasks is still rife in the population at large. In one study of doctors with children under ten years of age, two-thirds of male doctors reported that their partner or spouse would look after a child if he or she was ill on a school day, whereas only 2% of women had a partner or spouse who could do this. The rest of the women doctors mainly had to arrange for someone else other than themselves to care for the sick child.[10]

There is always a danger that the excellent childcare arrangements you thought you had made for your children will break down and you might end up putting them at risk (*see* Box 8.12).

Box 8.12:

When our au pair was delayed from returning from her holiday break back in Austria because of family illness, we thought it was time that we trusted our nine-year-old, Will, to come home alone from school, which is just down the road from our house. We had a key cut specially so that he could be a 'latch-key kid'. My GP surgery is only about 100 yards away from our house, so I could be there in a flash if there were any problems.

The first day went fine, but on the second, Will decided to make himself a sandwich and in doing so cut his thumb with the bread knife. He phoned me but I couldn't leave the surgery, and I ended up instructing him on how to bandage up his cut so that he could wait until I got home.

About half of the children whom we questioned thought that one of the benefits of having a doctor as a parent was that they took good medical care of you and others in your family. However, almost all of them thought that their doctor–parent often did not notice when they or others in the family were ill.

Sometimes it may be just the same as in any other family – a child is ill, and the parent assesses them and decides whether to send them to school or keep them at home. If both parents work and childcare is difficult, the child may feel that they have to be far more ill than some other children in order to get time off school (*see* Box 8.13).

Box 8.13:

Katie is seven years old. She loves the fact that her Mum is a doctor. She says that if anyone was ever sick in a plane or train, her Mum would be able to help. She often sees people come up to her Mum in the street and thank her for all her help, and that makes her feel proud that she can be recognised as her daughter.

However, Katie is at the age when she does not always want to go to school, perhaps because of the mental maths test, or because she has not learned her spellings that day. Any normal child can get away with putting talcum powder on their face or sticking their head against the hot radiator for as long as they can stand it. But not Katie. Her mother knows exactly when her daughter is truly ill. Even when she is feeling a bit unwell, Katie says that her Mum still normally packs her off to school after giving her a couple of teaspoons of paracetamol. She doesn't like always having to go to school when her friends' mothers always seem to let them off for the day in similar circumstances. That's the only thing that she can possibly see that's wrong with being a doctor's daughter – you simply have to learn your spellings on time.

On the other hand, some children are glad that the fact that their parent is a doctor means it is easier to obtain prompt medical treatment and they do not have to go trailing off to a doctor's surgery about minor illnesses (*see* Box 8.14).

Box 8.14:

If I'm feeling unwell then I don't have to make an appointment and go and see the doctor because Mum normally knows what's wrong with me. That can be a bad thing too, I suppose, because she always knows when I'm faking!

(Gaz, aged 16)

When a member of the family consults another doctor or health professional

When a child goes to see another doctor or health professional who knows their medical parent, they may find that they are not the centre of attention as they had a right to expect. The medic or nurse whom they are consulting may seem to be more interested in chatting about their doctor–parent instead of the child's ailment or needs (*see* Box 8.15).

Box 8.15:

Jamie is 15 years old. He attends a private school, which he admits he likes, even if there is too much work! Jamie is a keen rugby player and is in the school team. Last week he was injured during a match, and he now has to go and see the school nurse frequently for dressings. Jamie feels that whenever he goes to see the nurse, she is always more interested in what his Dad has been up to, as they used to work in the same department at the hospital many years ago. Despite the fact that he has to repeat himself to her every time he goes for treatment, she still asks after his father. He doesn't like this, as he feels that the nurse is more interested in his father than in him, and he should be the more important one – after all, he is injured, and it is her job to make him better.

A few of Jamie's other teachers used to be or still are his Dad's patients, and they have often spoken about him, too. He doesn't mind this as much, as they don't ask frequent questions like the school nurse, but he does object to the fact that at parents' evenings most of the allocated ten minutes that the parents have with some teachers is spent on the teacher's medical history. Jamie thinks that the staff at his school should remember that *he* is the person they should be most interested in, as they are being paid for this.

Sometimes it can be embarrassing for a child to consult a doctor or nurse who knows their mother or father, especially if they are a teenager with a personal problem or issue (*see* Box 8.16). They may fear that the doctor or nurse whom they are consulting will tell their parents what they have been up to, or what their innermost secrets or fears are. The scenario described in Box 8.16 can happen with any medical problem that a doctor's child may face. The child may end up feeling too embarrassed to go to the doctor to have their problems checked out.

Box 8.16:

Laura is 14 years old and has been in a relationship with her boyfriend for many months, and now she would like to take it to what she considers to be the next level. She and her boyfriend both made the decision together that they are going to sleep with each other, as they both agreed after talking about it that the risks of pregnancy were not applicable to them. However, something went wrong. What could she do?

After confiding in a friend they decided that the best option was to go to the doctor or family planning clinic. There was only one major problem that she

continued opposite

---

had to face that most other worried teenagers don't – her father was a well-known doctor, and she knew that she would be recognised as soon as she went in. She thought back to the last time she went to see her GP, which was quite a while ago, when she went about an infected eye. Even then he took one look at her name and address and immediately knew who she was, as he told her about when he had seen her father at some doctors' event. At the time she wasn't bothered and she really did not take much notice. Now she was faced with a different story, and she didn't dare to go and see him, as how was she to know that the confidentiality code was really kept? At her young age it would take a lot to place her trust in someone when she was feeling so vulnerable. She knew that if her family found out it would cause major problems, and that their views about her would completely change.

The major decision that she faced was whether to risk going to the doctor or to the family planning clinic, as the clinic staff might have connections with her father, too. She had to weigh up the alternatives and the risk of the doctor telling her father, or other doctors hearing about her consultation and in turn telling him, against the risk of not seeking medical advice at all.

Coping with serious illness in the family

A myriad of emotions arise when a doctor is faced with a partner, child or parent who is seriously ill. One common problem is that the doctor, who is already upset about seeing their loved one suffering and ill, is forced into the role of doctor, either directly administering care (*see* Box 8.17) or indirectly obtaining it (*see* Box 8.18).

Box 8.17:

Marg, a GP, had had a very close relationship with her father and was upset to watch him deteriorating slowly as his prostate cancer took hold.

A sudden crisis arose while Marg and her family were on holiday with her father. Her father developed urinary retention over a couple of days, and Marg decided to break off their holiday and move him to her home. Arriving home at midnight, she was reluctant to call a doctor out or take her father to the local Accident and Emergency department for an uncomfortable wait. So both of them agreed that the most convenient solution was for Marg to catheterise her father, which she did. The catheterisation went well and her father was very relieved. Breaching the child–parent taboo of the daughter undertaking such an intimate act was difficult for both of them, but it seemed to Marg to be justified on the basis of prioritising her father's comfort.

Box 8.18:

Andrew was shocked to find out that his wife's limp was due to multiple sclerosis. As the months went by the treating neurologist recommended interferon, but the hospital had no funding for his wife's treatment. As a doctor, Andrew was able to obtain supplies of the drug from overseas at a lower price that he could just about afford, despite being reduced to being a one-income family, and he could thus maintain his wife on treatment.[11]

If the medical or nursing care that the person who is ill receives is perceived by the rest of the family to be suboptimal, their relative who is also a doctor elsewhere may be forced to defend other health professionals, or be urged by the family to intervene. Box 8.19 demonstrates the conflicts that the dual professional and personal roles can cause.

Box 8.19: Daughter and doctor: two conflicting roles[12]

A GP working in London described her experience of her dual roles as daughter and doctor while her father was seriously ill.

'The most difficult aspect for me about my father's illness – dementia – is accessing my feelings about what is happening. My training as a doctor has made it hard for me to engage emotionally with what should otherwise be a time of grieving. I am slowly losing my father and yet I struggle to find any tears ...

I find myself in constant conflict about my roles as daughter and doctor. As I write, we are waiting for a bed for him in a specialist hospital, and there is nothing I can do to make one materialise faster. I find myself rationalising the situation to the family – this is how the service works, and his own doctors have it under control. My mother asks me to intervene, to see if I can speed things up – I am, after all, a doctor. Eventually we hear that they have decided that moving my father will not achieve anything, and I'm inclined to agree ...

My father finally saw a neurologist and got his diagnosis. The GP would not prescribe the medication that was suggested by the neurologist. He said he was not willing to take responsibility for it. With a heavy heart at such a blurring of my roles I agreed to provide the prescriptions myself ...'

Some solutions

Confidentiality

Every effort should be made to ensure that confidentiality is not breached for a doctor or a member of their family consulting the health service, just as for anyone else. This may mean providing alternative arrangements so that a sick doctor is not being treated alongside their usual patients (*see* Box 8.20).

Box 8.20:

When Mick, a well-known consultant physician, became seriously depressed, the local psychiatrist liaised with a colleague in another county and Mick was admitted to a psychiatric hospital where no one except for essential medical and nursing staff knew that he was a doctor.

This made it much easier for Mick to return to work once he had recovered. Only close colleagues whom he had told himself knew the reason for his sickness absence.

Confidentiality is difficult but possible to preserve in a small tight-knit community where the doctors' children or other family members are well known. Discuss the possible problems with regard to preserving confidentiality as a team in your practice or workplace. How will notes be stored securely? Is everyone aware of the confidentiality policy? Undertake a significant event audit of any breach of confidentiality that does occur in order to pinpoint where improvements can be made and ensure that your new systems mean that such a breach cannot be repeated.

Confidentiality may only be broken 'in the most exceptional situations when the health, safety or welfare of the patient, or others, would otherwise be at grave risk. The decision as to whether to break confidentiality depends on the degree of current or potential harm ...'[13] Young people should feel secure about the confidential nature of any consultation with a doctor or nurse.

Awareness of the doctor's child's perspective

At work, perhaps you can discuss the insights that the young people have given here about how it feels to be treated by a doctor or nurse who is more interested in chatting about their parent than about the child and the problem with which they are consulting.

At home, make more effort to actively listen to your child when they are telling you that they feel unwell or are seeking your help for their health-related problem. Take more time to explain why they do not need investigation or treatment, if you think that is the case, rather than brushing them aside and implying that they are wasting your time. Think hard before you offer an opinion or treat them, if in a non-medical home a parent would be taking them to see a doctor or nurse. Give your child the opportunity to consult an independent practitioner as a routine. Then they will know how to do so for themselves when they are teenagers.

References

1 Chambers R and Belcher J (1992) Self-reported health care over the past 10 years: a survey of general practitioners. *Br J Gen Pract.* **42**: 153–6.

2 Thompson W, Cupples M, Sibbett C *et al.* (2001) Challenge of culture, conscience and contract to general practitioners' care of their own health: qualitative study. *BMJ.* **323**: 728–31.

3 McKevitt C, Morgan M, Dundas R *et al.* (1997) Sickness absence and 'working through' illness: a comparison of two professional groups. *J Pub Health Med.* **19**: 295–300.

4 Lindeman S, Laara E, Hakko H *et al.* (1996) A systematic review of gender-specific suicide mortality in medical doctors. *Br J Psychiatry.* **168**: 274–9.

5 British Medical Association (1998) *Working Group on the Misuse of Alcohol and Drugs by Doctors.* British Medical Association, London.

6 British Medical Association (1995) *Guidelines for Ethical Responsibilities in Treating Doctor–Patients.* British Medical Association, London.

7 Pattani S, Constantinovici N and Williams S (2001) Who retires early from the NHS because of ill health and what does it cost? A national cross-sectional study. *BMJ.* **322**: 208–9.

8 Chambers R and Belcher J (1994) Predicting mental health problems in general practitioners. *Occup Med.* **44**: 212–6.

9 Chambers R and Campbell I (1996) Anxiety and depression in general practitioners: associations with type of practice, fundholding, gender and other personal characteristics. *Fam Pract.* **13**: 170–3.

10 Chambers R and Campbell I (1996) Gender differences in general practitioners at work. *Br J Gen Pract.* **46**: 291–3.

11 Dyson A (2001) The price isn't right. *BMJ.* **323**: 407.

12 Anon. (2002) Daughter and doctor: two conflicting roles. *BMJ.* **324**: 1530.

13 Donovan C, Hadley A, Jones M *et al.* (2000) *Confidentiality and Young People Toolkit.* Royal College of General Practitioners, London.

9

Surviving as a doctor's family: making a logical plan

This book is packed full of good advice. You will have heard a considerable amount of it before. You know what you should do – but you haven't put that good advice into practice. Something crops up to distract you from setting your plans in motion to improve your home life or work–home balance. You mean to spend more time with your spouse or partner, but your good intentions do not last for long. You enjoy your holiday and vow to take the children out to all kinds of activities in future, but when you are back at work you soon become tired and preoccupied again.

Does this sound familiar? You need to reflect on why your good resolutions to improve your marital/family life have failed in the past. It is probably because *carrying out* your resolution was a lot more complex a matter than simply making the resolution. Other factors may have intruded that you had not foreseen. Your will-power might not have been sufficient, you may not have had the skills, time or money for your new promised way of life, or you may have mistakenly assumed that others would support you in making your planned changes.

You could regard reducing and managing the stresses and pressures in your family life as a project and use the logical framework (log-frame) approach to help you to succeed in carrying out your good resolutions. This type of project management approach sets out the activities, achievements and purpose with regard to achieving your goal(s). The log frame handles the complex nature of making and undertaking an action plan to improve all of the dimensions of your life and set specific goal(s). It helps you to analyse your weaknesses and guides you to consider the assumptions that you are making – in the details of your action plan or in pursuing your goals. This approach helps you to recognise the interactions between what you can do for yourself and the external factors that either enhance or hinder your plans.

The log frame helps you to set out realistic milestones and to decide in advance how you will monitor your progress. It helps you to:

- organise your thinking
- relate your planned activities to the results you can expect

- set performance indicators for yourself
- allocate responsibilities for yourself and to others – both at work and at home.

Advantages of a logical framework

The logical framework has been used for project planning for decades.[1] Development agencies have adopted the approach for planning and monitoring overseas programmes, and recently it has been used by the health service for planning and evaluating Health Action Zone projects.[2,3]

The approach will force you to consider the assumptions that you are making in setting out your action plan. You will be able to monitor your progress and pre-empt obstructions to your plans. The log frame is an aid to thinking rather than a series of procedures to which you should slavishly adhere. The framework will help you to concentrate on the operational aspects of your survival 'project' and on who is doing what to whom, when, why and how.[1]

The structure of the log frame is a 4×4 matrix (*see* Table 9.1). The rows represent the project objectives and the means of achieving them (*vertical logic*). The columns indicate how you can verify that you have achieved your objectives (*horizontal logic*) and the assumptions that you are making.

Table 9.1: Simple 4×4 matrix of a logical framework			
Summary	*Indicators*	*Verification*	*Assumptions*
Goal			
Purpose			
Outcomes (intermediate achievements)			
Activities			

We have adapted the log-frame approach to help you to undertake your personal project on surviving and thriving both as a doctor and as a family. (If you want to look at another related but different example considering stress at work in a health setting, you can see how a goal stated as 'To minimise stress in my working life' works out in Chambers R, Schwartz A and Boath E (2003) *Beating Stress in the NHS.* Radcliffe Medical Press, Oxford.)

The vertical logic

- *Step 1*. Define your overall *goal* – the reason for you undertaking the 'project'. This is the ultimate objective of your survival programme. Phrase this in your own words. An example might be *to achieve a happy home life*. You might choose to set an entirely different goal and that is what you ultimately seek.
- *Step 2*. Define the *purpose* of the 'project'. The purpose is why you are proposing to carry out the project – what it will achieve once it is completed within your timescale, and what impact you hope to make. It is the motivation behind the outcomes of the project (*see* Step 3). An example might be *to have a sensible work–home balance*. It keeps the project more streamlined if you only have one purpose. Although you will try your best, it will not be entirely within your control to achieve the purpose of your project. In the example given here, you might be unable to influence all of the family to join in your proposed changes, even though you and others have undertaken the preliminary work that demonstrates the need.
- *Step 3*. Define the *outcomes* for achieving the purpose of the 'project'. These are what you want the project to achieve – the specific end results that will be achieved when the planned activities are carried out. We have called them 'intermediate achievements' in Table 9.1, as they are on the way to gaining your purpose and thereafter your overall goal. An example might be *to be competent in assertiveness skills*. Achieving the outcomes should be within your control.
- *Step 4*. Define the *activities* that you will undertake in order to achieve each outcome, and what resources are available. Activities define how you will carry out your project. Examples might be to *keep a log of how you spend your time* or *attend assertiveness training*. You should expect to undertake three to seven activities for every outcome you hope to accomplish (*see* Table 9.3 for an example).

The log-frame structure is based on the concept of cause and effect. The vertical logic is based on a sequence of causal relationships starting from the bottom upwards. There is a logical relationship between activities and outcomes, outcomes and the purpose, and the purpose and the goal. Therefore *if* specific activities are carried out *then* certain outcomes will be produced. If the outcomes you describe are produced, then the declared purpose will be achieved. If the purpose is achieved, your goal should be attained.

So from the bottom upwards:

GOAL

then ↑

if PURPOSE

then ↑

if OUTCOMES

then ↑

if ACTIVITIES

Evaluate your results sequentially, from the bottom upwards. You cannot logically evaluate the *outcomes* of your activities without first monitoring whether the *activities* have been carried out and achieved as planned. Similarly, you cannot expect to obtain the improvements described in your *purpose* without the *outcomes* having been achieved first.

The horizontal logic

Horizontal logic underlies the way in which you measure the effectiveness of your plan. Specify how you will measure progress for each of the four levels of the vertical logic – the activities, outcomes, purpose and goal. As far as possible, use concrete terms rather than vague measures as tangible indicators of progress. These indicators should have the following qualities.

*   They clearly describe how the achievement of the activity, outcome or purpose contributes to the success of the project.
*   They focus on what is important for the purpose or overall goal.
*   They clearly relate to the activity, outcome, purpose or goal with which they are associated.
*   They are of sufficient number and detailed enough to measure activities, outcomes, purpose and goal adequately.
*   They are specific to an activity, outcome, purpose or goal.
*   They are objectively verifiable, so that two independent observers measure achievement in the same way – whether quantitative or qualitative in nature.

The indicator might be direct (e.g. number of days' holiday you spend together in a year) or indirect (e.g. your own or your family's sporting or hobby achievements).

These indicators, like others elsewhere, should be *SMART*:

- **S**pecific
- **M**easurable
- **A**chievable
- **R**ealistic
- **T**ime-limited.

Then decide how you will verify that all of the specified indicators have been achieved. You might gather simple data as part of your project, or refer to sources of information such as reports, surveys, official documents, notes of meetings or a review of case studies over time.

'For each level of the vertical logic there will be a set of objectively verifiable indicators which are appropriate to the objectives at that level and which constitute proof of achievement at that level'.[1]

Important assumptions

You know that it is very unlikely that your plans will go forward without a hitch, but that doesn't stop you assuming that you will progress smoothly. In reality, unexpected things crop up which obstruct or delay your progress.

The assumptions that you describe in your log frame include factors or conditions that could affect your progress with the project or its overall success, over which you have no or only limited control. For the overseas development projects with which the log frame has been used, these might include external factors such as unexpected bad weather or an earthquake.

For you, trying to achieve a happy home life, examples of major external factors that are beyond your control might include the illness of your partner/spouse or a member of the family, or a sick colleague at work necessitating your working longer hours. More minor external factors might include the extent of co-operation that is forthcoming from others in your family or your colleagues at work if you are proposing to reduce your working hours. These will affect whether you are able to undertake many of the activities you plan, or to achieve the outcomes or purpose in your log frame.

As well as the unexpected factors that might spoil your plans, you may be assuming too much. It may be that you and others in your family have insufficient knowledge and skills to carry out the activities that you envisage, or you might not have forecast the extent of time or income needed to implement your plans.

There may be other risks to your planned timetable, too. You may not have thought through the consequences of your plans (e.g. how you will manage on less income to be in line with your plans). Or you may not have predicted the new stress-provoking factors which might arise from the revised weekly schedule (perhaps spending more time together at home will provoke arguments rather than boost happiness as you had hoped).

Getting started

Read through the series of steps below and work through the thinking behind the way in which we have put the log frame together. Before you start, note down all of the people who will have some influence on the progress or viability of your family survival plan throughout the lifetime of your 'project'. They might include the following:

- your spouse/partner at home
- your family
- friends with whom you socialise or play sport
- colleagues at work
- managers in your department, practice or trust
- staff at work to whom you delegate tasks
- people who delegate work to you
- people for whom you are responsible
- your cleaner or gardener at home
- relatives who are dependent on you, etc.

You will need to anticipate how they will influence your plan – to enhance or limit progress. So consider how they will interact with you and include them in the activities of your log frame, or in the assumptions that you make. You will be taking account of their influence – by harnessing their help or preventing them from obstructing you – in the nature of the activities that you include in your plan.

The worked example that we shall develop below illustrates the processes that you need to adopt to make up a log frame. The contents of the example log frame are an illustration of the thinking behind a log frame, and are not prescriptive. You should use the evolving framework as a guide, rather than lift the example 'off the peg' for your own requirements. Much of the learning and benefits from a log frame arise from the preparatory work involved in putting it together and thinking through the factors that are individual to you and which will enhance or prevent your progress. They will be unique to you, your family and networks of contacts and your circumstances.

We have not included every detail of the possible assumptions or potential risks that might occur during such a project plan, or even the numerous activities that you could undertake. To do so would have resulted in such a vast amount of background detail that it would be difficult for the reader to distinguish 'must do' information from 'could do' detail. You will be able to include more information about risks and assumptions yourself. The columns of a completed log frame that is undertaken over a period of a year or more often stretch to over three or four sides of A4 paper.[4]

Have a first go at establishing the vertical logic.

- *Step 1*. Have a go at writing down the goal of your 'project'. In Table 9.2, this is *to achieve a happy home life*. You might want to take a wider view and consider that your ultimate goal is to be a much happier person at work and at home.
- *Step 2*. Have a go at writing down the purpose of your 'project'. In Table 9.2, this is *to have a sensible work–home balance*.
- *Step 3*. Have a go at writing down the outcomes of your 'project' that, taken together, will achieve your purpose. These are really intermediate achievements in your progress plan. In Table 9.2, these are *competent in assertiveness skills, protected time for activities outside work* and *good relationships with partner, family and friends*. Now you need to challenge yourself. Are there gaps? Are these three outcomes appropriate for your purpose?
- *Step 4*. Have a go at writing down the activities that you initially think might achieve each outcome. In Table 9.2, these include (in brief) *attend assertiveness training course, keep a log of how you spend your time, review sources of stress in home life* and *hold family meeting*.

Now you should apply the 'If–then' logic described previously to test out the cause-and-effect relationship. *If* these activities are carried out, *then* you will achieve these outcomes. *If* you attend a training course on assertiveness, *then*

Table 9.2: Step 1 of building up the log frame to thrive as a happy medical family: your first attempt at planning your vertical logical pathway

	Summary	*Indicators*	*Verification*	*Assumptions*
Goal	**To achieve a happy home life**			
Purpose	**To have a sensible work–home balance**			
Outcomes (intermediate achievements)	**Competent in assertiveness skills** **Protected time for activities outside work** **Good relationships with partner, family and friends**			
Activities	**Attend assertiveness training course** **Keep a timed activity log of activities at work and outside work** **Review sources of stress at home from perspectives of self and partner/family** **Convene family meeting to discuss problems and changes everyone wishes to make**			

you will be competent in assertiveness. You can see that the case is crumbling – there are missing links.

You will have to do more than simply attend an assertiveness training course. You will have to practise being assertive to become competent and improve with feedback from others about your assertiveness technique. You have been assuming that attending a training course is all that you need to do, whereas in fact in addition to activities such as practising the skills you have learned you should have undertaken linked activities, such as prioritising learning about assertiveness skills, located an appropriate training course, setting aside time to go, justifying the course fees, etc.

Look again at these activities and outcomes. *If* you review your stressors at home and keep a log of how you spend your time, *then* … what? The outcomes described in Table 9.2 were about finding protected time for activities outside work and establishing good relationships with your partner, family and friends. There are *no* intermediate steps in the list of activities for converting the information gathered in the review of how you spend your time to controlling the sources of stress identified or protecting time for leisure activities, and *no* specific outcomes for each activity, so you need to add some more activities, as we do **in bold** in Table 9.3.

Numbering the outcomes and the activities linked to them will help you to see how *if* you undertake certain activities *then* you will achieve specific outcomes, as in Table 9.3.

Now that you are beginning to get the vertical logic in place, you should start thinking out what assumptions you have been making, and if there are any potential risks associated with your logical plan. Once you have recognised these, you may have to add in other activities in order to minimise the effects of previously unforeseen external factors. This is the stage when you should be anticipating problems that could interrupt the progress of your project action plan. You may have a blind spot about these possible problem areas, so you could usefully discuss the preliminary thinking of your project plan with someone else, such as your partner or a friend, who might point out weaknesses that you have not yet recognised, or give you information about possible external influences of which you were unaware.

The additions **in bold** in Table 9.4 provide some examples of assumptions that you might be making. You can see that as you think through how you are going to undertake these activities and turn them into outcomes, some gaps are appearing – you may be assuming that you already possess the knowledge and skills necessary to draw up a personal development plan, or that you are capable of undertaking a review of sources of stress at home. The next step is to add more activities to the Summary column in order to address these assumptions, as we do later in Table 9.5.

The type of *risks* that may arise include the following: you waste your time attending an assertiveness skills course that does not fit your needs; you identify topics that you urgently need to learn more about, and you therefore cannot

Table 9.3: Step 2 of building up the log frame to thrive as a happy medical family: linking activities with outputs

	Summary	Indicators	Verification	Assumptions
Goal	To achieve a happy home life			
Purpose	To have a sensible work–home balance			
Outcomes (intermediate achievements)	1 Competent in assertiveness skills 2 Protected time for activities outside work 3 Good relationships with partner, family and friends			
Activities	**1.1 Draw up a personal development plan (PDP) and prioritise assertiveness** **1.2 Arrange to learn about assertiveness; find resources to provide cover and course fee, locate training course** 1.3 Attend assertiveness training course **1.4 Practise assertiveness with family and colleagues; obtain feedback from both** 2.1 Keep a timed activity log of activities at work and outside work **2.2 Discuss time/activities log with colleagues at work and family at home. Make a plan for non-work activities** **2.3 Join a health club and attend induction** **2.4 Review personal and professional diaries and write in non-work activities** 2.5 Review sources of stress at home from perspectives of self and partner/family **2.6 Discuss stressors and job satisfaction with partner at home** 3.1 Convene family meeting to discuss problems and changes everyone wishes to make **3.2 Invite friends round for a series of meals, outings** **3.3 Review own and partner's work commitments and career aspirations together** **3.4 Conduct audit of own job satisfaction**			

Table 9.4: Step 3 of building up the log frame to thrive as a happy medical family: adding in assumptions about your planned activities

	Summary	Indicators	Verification	Assumptions
Goal	1 To achieve a happy home life			
Purpose	1 To have a sensible work–home balance			
Outcomes (intermediate achievements)	1 Competent in assertiveness skills 2 Protected time for activities outside work 3 Good relationships with partner, family and friends			
Activities	1.1 Draw up a PDP and prioritise assertiveness 1.2 Arrange to learn about assertiveness; find resources to provide cover and course fee, locate training course 1.3 Attend assertiveness training course 1.4 Practise assertiveness with family and colleagues; obtain feedback from both 2.1 Keep a timed activity log of activities at work and outside work 2.2 Discuss time/activities log with colleagues at work and family at home. Make a plan for non-work activities 2.3 Join a health club and attend induction 2.4 Review personal and professional diaries and write in non-work activities			**1.1 You know how to draw up a PDP/ identify learning needs** **1.2 Resources will be forthcoming; course will be accessible and available** **1.3 Assertiveness can be learned by attending a training course** **1.4 Practising on family and colleagues prepares you for the real world; you can become competent within the timescale of the project plan** **2.1 You have the time and skills to organise a workload and time/ activities survey** **2.2 Colleagues and family will be interested and willing to help** **2.3 A health club is local to you; the health club ambience appeals to you** **2.4 Commitments already made allow inclusion of non-work activities; you are assertive enough with yourself to prioritise non-work activities**

Table 9.4: Continued

Summary	Indicators	Verification	Assumptions
2.5 Review sources of stress at home from perspectives of self and partner/family			**2.5 You are sufficiently skilled in identifying sources of stress from different perspectives**
2.6 Discuss stressors and job satisfaction with partner at home			**2.6 You have a partner; your partner is willing to listen**
3.1 Convene family meeting to discuss problems and changes everyone wishes to make			**3.1 All of your family members are willing to become engaged**
3.2 Invite friends round for a series of meals, outings			**3.2 Friends exist; friends who do exist are willing to be engaged**
3.3 Review own and partner's work commitments and career aspirations together			**3.3 You (and your partner) have kept an activity log and are willing to review log in a constructive manner; you (and partner) have reflected on career aspirations, know of career opportunities and can discuss important plans together**
3.4 Conduct audit of own job satisfaction			**3.4 You have skills to undertake audit; you have knowledge of sources of job satisfaction in general and relevant to you**

justify learning more about assertiveness; you cannot find the right course pitched at an appropriate level for you, that is held at a convenient time and is affordable. Other areas of risk will include the following: staff numbers remain stable; no significant new Government directives are issued that overturn your priorities at work; no crisis occurs at your workplace (e.g. a flood or fire).

So the next step is to add yet more activities to anticipate the risks that you realise could happen, and to reduce the likelihood of them occurring and obstructing your progress with your plan. The risks and activities shown **in bold** in Table 9.5 illustrate a variety of risks that might occur and activities that you might adopt in order to minimise the effects of these risks on your progress towards achieving a happier and more balanced life.

The next step is to move on to specify the assumptions that you are making about achieving your outcomes. Examples of these have been added **in bold** in Table 9.6.

For instance, you may assume that you can protect time for leisure activities in a regular way, whereas in reality there will be unforeseen circumstances that interrupt your plans. There will be a potential risk, for example, that in protecting time for a special new interest for yourself, new time pressures are created for the rest of the family that are at least as bad as the original situation. The family discussions which you have already added as an activity might be an opportunity to discuss ways in which the family as a whole, rather than just you, can achieve a less pressured and happier home life.

Now it is time to map out the assumptions and risks associated with your purpose and overall goal. We have started this process in the additions shown **in bold** in Table 9.7 below, but in reality you would have far more to add to these sections. You need to think of any external factors that are required, or that might prevent the long-term sustainability of your goal or purpose, for the project to be successful.

You will also need to think about the 'potential risks' that are likely to arise. The assumptions that you are making and the risks you anticipate should trigger you to add extra activities and outcomes to your right-hand column in real life. We have *not* added any extra activities or outcomes here (to anticipate assumptions and risks of the purpose and goal in our example log frame in Table 9.7) for the sake of simplicity, but you will certainly have to do so in order to take adequate measures to ensure smooth progress with your plan.

Your final step will be to describe the indicators for all of your activities, outcomes, purpose and goal, as well as the means by which you can verify that you have achieved them. You should add a timescale, too, for each indicator. The indicators should be achievable and worthwhile. Turn back to page 108 to remind yourself of the ideal characteristics of indicators.

The examples added to Table 9.8 are shown **in bold.** They illustrate how someone might do their best to fix appropriate indicators and give examples of how the indicators might be verified.

Table 9.5: Step 4 of building up the log frame to thrive as a happy medical family: adding in more activities to anticipate the risks' that may arise from previously planned activities and assumptions

	Summary	Indicators	Verification	Assumptions and risks
Goal	1 To achieve a happy home life			
Purpose	1 To have a sensible work–home balance			
Outcomes (intermediate achievements)	1 Competent in assertiveness skills 2 Protected time for activities outside work 3 Good relationships with partner, family and friends			
Activities	1.1 Draw up a PDP and prioritise assertiveness 1.2 Arrange to learn about assertiveness; find resources to provide cover and course fee, locate training course 1.3 Attend assertiveness training course 1.4 Practise assertiveness with family and colleagues; obtain feedback from both **1.5 Obtain course curriculum and talk to someone who has been to the proposed assertiveness training course to find out more about it** 2.1 Keep a timed activity log of activities at work and outside work 2.2 Discuss time/activities log with colleagues at work and family at home. Make a plan for non-work activities 2.3 Join a health club and attend induction			*Assumptions* 1.1 You know how to draw up a PDP/identify learning needs 1.2 Resources will be forthcoming; course will be accessible and available 1.3 Assertiveness can be learned by attending a training course 1.4 Practising on family and colleagues prepares you for the real world; you can become competent within the timescale of the project plan *Risks* **1.5 Assertiveness course is inappropriate for you** *Assumptions* 2.1 You have the time and skills to organise a workload and time/activities survey 2.2 Colleagues and family will be interested and willing to help 2.3 A health club is local to you; the health club ambience appeals to you

Table 9.5: Continued

	Summary	Indicators	Verification	Assumptions and risks
	2.4 Review personal and professional diaries and write in non-work activities			2.4 Commitments already made allow inclusion of non-work activities; you are assertive enough with yourself to prioritise non-work activities
	2.5 Review sources of stress at home from perspectives of self and partner/family			2.5 You are sufficiently skilled in identifying sources of stress from different perspectives
	2.6 Discuss stressors and job satisfaction with partner at home			2.6 You have a partner; your partner is willing to listen
				Risks
	2.7 Visit several health clubs and try sample days before joining one as member			**2.7 You do not like the ethos of the health club and rarely go**
	2.8 Agree a rota with siblings to help parent who is ill			**2.8 One of your parents becomes increasingly ill and you have to spend non-work time helping them**
	3.1 Convene family meeting to discuss problems and changes everyone wishes to make			3.1 All your family members are willing to become engaged
	3.2 Invite friends round for a series of meals, outings			3.2 Friends exist; friends who do exist are willing to be engaged
	3.3 Review own and partner's work commitments and career aspirations together			3.3 You (and your partner) have kept an activity log and are willing to review log in a constructive manner; you (and partner) have reflected on career aspirations, know of career opportunities and can discuss important plans together
	3.4 Conduct audit of own job satisfaction			3.4 You have skills to undertake audit; you have knowledge of sources of job satisfaction in general and relevant to you
				Risks
	3.5 Arrangements for meetings with partner and family to discuss changes optimise their attendance (e.g. with dinner or promise of outing afterwards)			**3.5 Member(s) of family cancel meeting you arrange to discuss family matters, as time with their friends takes precedence**

Table 9.6: Step 5 of building up the log frame to thrive as a happy medical family: adding assumptions that you are making about expected outcomes and adding more activities to reduce the likelihood of potential risks occurring

	Summary	Indicators	Verification	Assumptions and risks
Goal	1 To achieve a happy home life			
Purpose	1 To have a sensible work–home balance			
Outcomes (intermediate achievements)	1 Competent in assertiveness skills			*Assumptions* 1.1 **You apply your new knowledge and skills in assertiveness consistently, whatever the provocation**
	2 Protected time for activities outside work			2.1 **Your weekly schedule is typical and does not have unforeseen 'crises' that disrupt it** 2.2 **You have activities outside work that you enjoy**
	3 Good relationships with partner, family and friends			3.1 **All positively want to make relationships work** 3.2 **All have time to make good relationships happen** *Risks* 3.2 **Life event occurs (bereavement, friends or family move away, older relative moves in)**
Activities	1.1 Draw up a PDP and prioritise assertiveness			*Assumptions* 1.1 You know how to draw up a PDP/identify learning needs
	1.2 Arrange to learn about assertiveness; find resources to provide cover and course fee, locate training course			1.2 Resources will be forthcoming; course will be accessible and available
	1.3 Attend assertiveness training course			1.3 Assertiveness can be learned by attending a training course

Table 9.6: Continued

Summary	Indicators	Verification	Assumptions and risks
1.4 Practise assertiveness with family and colleagues; obtain feedback from both			1.4 Practising on family and colleagues prepares you for the real world; you can become competent within the timescale of the project plan
			Risks
1.5 Obtain course curriculum and talk to someone who has been to the proposed assertiveness training course to find out more about it			1.5 Assertiveness course is inappropriate for you
			Assumptions
2.1 Keep a timed activity log of activities at work and outside work			2.1 You have the time and skills to organise a workload and time/activities survey
2.2 Discuss time/activities log with colleagues at work and family at home. Make a plan for non-work activities			2.2 Colleagues and family will be interested and willing to help
2.3 Join a health club and attend induction			2.3 A health club is local to you; the health club ambience appeals to you
2.4 Review personal and professional diaries and write in non-work activities			2.4 Commitments already made allow inclusion of non-work activities; you are assertive enough with yourself to prioritise non-work activities
2.5 Review sources of stress at home from perspectives of self and partner/family			2.5 You are sufficiently skilled in identifying sources of stress from different perspectives
2.6 Discuss stressors and job satisfaction with partner at home			2.6 You have a partner; your partner is willing to listen
			Risks
2.7 Visit several health clubs and try sample days before joining one as member			2.7 You do not like the ethos of the health club and rarely go
2.8 Agree a rota with siblings to help parent who is ill			2.8 One of your parents becomes increasingly ill and you have to spend non-work time helping them

Table 9.6: Continued

Summary	Indicators	Verification	Assumptions and risks
2.9 Take up new hobby you have always intended to pursue			**2.9 The time taken up by new hobby may create new pressures on family life**
			Assumptions
3.1 Convene family meeting to discuss problems and changes everyone wishes to make			3.1 All your family members are willing to become engaged
3.2 Invite friends round for a series of meals, outings			3.2 Friends exist; friends who do exist are willing to be engaged
3.3 Review own and partner's work commitments and career aspirations together			3.3 You (and your partner) have kept an activity log and are willing to review log in a constructive manner; you (and partner) have reflected on career aspirations, know of career opportunities and can discuss important plans together
3.4 Conduct audit of own job satisfaction			3.4 You have skills to undertake audit; you have knowledge of sources of job satisfaction in general and relevant to you
			Risks
3.5 Arrangements for meetings with partner and family to discuss changes optimise their attendance (e.g. with dinner or promise of outing afterwards)			3.5 Member(s) of family cancel meeting you arrange to discuss family matters, as time with their friends takes precedence

Table 9.7: Step 6 of building up the log frame to thrive as a happy medical family: adding various assumptions that you are making about your purpose and goal

	Summary	Indicators	Verification	Assumptions and risks
Goal	1 To achieve a happy home life			*Assumptions* 1.1 You remain working (in the post of your plan) 1.2 You and your family remain in good health *Risks* 1.3 Other significant life events occur 1.4 Your job no longer exists due to NHS changes
Purpose	1 To have a sensible work–home balance			*Assumptions* 1.1 You revise your current post in the way you desire, or you find a new post that meets your requirements 1.2 You have the resources to control sources of stress at home and at work 1.3 The planned stress management is effective in reducing stress for you and your family and building good relationships 1.4 You preserve the protected time that you build into your weekly schedule for yourself – keeping fit and hobbies; for your partner – communicating; for your family – sharing activities *Risks* 1.5 You cannot meet the usual costs of your family on your new lower income from reduced working hours 1.6 Your family relationships are beyond repair

Table 9.7: Continued

	Summary	Indicators	Verification	Assumptions and risks
Outcomes (intermediate achievements)	1 Competent in assertiveness skills			Assumptions 1.1 You apply your new knowledge and skills in assertiveness consistently, whatever the provocation
	2 Protected time for activities outside work			2.1 Your weekly schedule is typical and does not have unforeseen 'crises' that disrupt it 2.2 You have activities outside work that you enjoy
	3 Good relationships with partner, family and friends			3.1 All positively want to make relationships work 3.2 All have time to make good relationships happen Risks 3.2 Life event occurs (bereavement, friends or family move away, older relative moves in)
Activities	1.1 Draw up a PDP and prioritise assertiveness			Assumptions 1.1 You know how to draw up a PDP/identify learning needs
	1.2 Arrange to learn about assertiveness; find resources to provide cover and course fee, locate training course			1.2 Resources will be forthcoming; course will be accessible and available
	1.3 Attend assertiveness training course			1.3 Assertiveness can be learned by attending a training course
	1.4 Practise assertiveness with family and colleagues; obtain feedback from both			1.4 Practising on family and colleagues prepares you for the real world; you can become competent within the timescale of the project plan

Table 9.7: Continued

Summary	Indicators	Verification	Assumptions and risks
1.5 Obtain course curriculum and talk to someone who has been to the proposed assertiveness training course to find out more about it			*Risks* 1.5 Assertiveness course is inappropriate for you
2.1 Keep a timed activity log of activities at work and outside work			*Assumptions* 2.1 You have the time and skills to organise a workload and time/activities survey
2.2 Discuss time/activities log with colleagues at work and family at home. Make plan for non-work activities			2.2 Colleagues and family will be interested and willing to help
2.3 Join a health club and attend induction			2.3 A health club is local to you; the health club ambience appeals to you
2.4 Review personal and professional diaries and write in non-work activities			2.4 Commitments already made allow inclusion of non-work activities; you are assertive enough with yourself to prioritise non-work activities
2.5 Review sources of stress at home from perspectives of self and partner/family			2.5 You are sufficiently skilled in identifying sources of stress from different perspectives
2.6 Discuss stressors and job satisfaction with partner at home			2.6 You have a partner; your partner is willing to listen
2.7 Visit several health clubs and try sample days before joining one as member			*Risks* 2.7 You do not like the ethos of the health club and rarely go
2.8 Agree a rota with siblings to help parent who is ill			2.8 One of your parents becomes increasingly ill and you have to spend non-work time helping them
2.9 Take up new hobby you have always intended to pursue			2.9 The time taken up by new hobby may create new pressures on family life

Table 9.7: Continued

Summary	Indicators	Verification	Assumptions and risks
3.1 Convene family meeting to discuss problems and changes everyone wishes to make			*Assumptions*
			3.1 All your family members are willing to become engaged
3.2 Invite friends round for a series of meals, outings			3.2 Friends exist; friends who do exist are willing to be engaged
3.3 Review own and partner's work commitments and career aspirations together			3.3 You (and your partner) have kept an activity log and are willing to review log in a constructive manner; you (and partner) have reflected on career aspirations, know of career opportunities and can discuss important plans together
3.4 Conduct audit of own job satisfaction			3.4 You have skills to undertake audit; you have knowledge of sources of job satisfaction in general and relevant to you
			Risks
3.5 Arrangements for meetings with partner and family to discuss changes optimise their attendance (e.g. with dinner or promise of outing afterwards)			3.5 Member(s) of family cancel meeting you arrange to discuss family matters, as time with their friends takes precedence

Table 9.8: Step 7 of building up the log frame to thrive as a happy medical family: adding indicators and the means of verification of progress for your planned activities, outcomes, purpose and goal (as examples here)

	Summary	Indicators (examples)	Verification (examples)	Assumptions and risks
Goal	1 To achieve a happy home life	**1 You and others have a feeling of well-being for majority of the time at home**	**1 Follow-up family review reveals that every member rates significant improvements in their own and others' home lives and can give tangible examples of this**	As for Table 9.7
Purpose	1 To have a sensible work–home balance	**1.1 Agreed milestones representing increased contentment levels in (i) partner, (ii) family and (iii) you at home and at work** **1.2 Agreed balance of time spent at work, on chores at home, or on fun/leisure – for you, partner and family**	**1.1 and 1.2 Follow-up review with your partner at home shows milestones reached and your expected coping methods are in place, and agreed extent of time for work, chores at home, fun/leisure have been met**	As for Table 9.7
Outcomes (intermediate achievements)	1 Competent in assertiveness skills 2 Protected time for activities outside work	**1.1 Act assertively with family and colleagues consistently after you have been on course** **2.1 Regular sport activities and hobbies in weekly schedule**	**1.1 Feedback about the extent of your assertiveness given at annual peer appraisal at work and in discussion with partner** **2.1 Your diary shows how you spent time on sport and hobbies at least three times a week, every week, in first six months**	As for Table 9.7

Table 9.8: Continued

	Summary	Indicators (examples)	Verification (examples)	Assumptions and risks
	3 Good relationships with partner, family and friends	**2.2 Learned to play musical instrument by one year**	**2.2 Good enough to play musical instrument with friends**	
		3.1 Every member of the family feels that they belong	**3.1 Discussion and attendance at regular family get-togethers shows this**	
		3.2 All members of family have a network of friends with whom they meet up regularly	**3.2 Every member of the family spends time (e.g. at least 3 hours a week) with friends outside work/ school**	
		3.3 Your relationship with partner lasts forever	**3.3 You do not get divorced or separate from your long-term partner/spouse; you have a regular sex life; you have regular discussions**	
Activities	1.1 Draw up a PDP and prioritise assertiveness	**1.1 PDP drawn up; learning needs prioritised**	**1.1 PDP approved at annual appraisal (each year) at work**	As for Table 9.7
	1.2 Arrange to learn about assertiveness; find resources to provide cover and course fee, locate training course	**1.2 Course booked by x months; bid for training budget for course fee**	**1.2 Application made; bid for course fee successful**	
	1.3 Attend assertiveness training course	**1.3 Attend course**	**1.3 Attend course**	
	1.4 Practise assertiveness with family and colleagues; obtain feedback from both	**1.4 Assertiveness skills used regularly with partner/ children at home and with colleagues at work**	**1.4 Significant event audit at work demonstrating assertiveness included in PDP; and similar review at home discussed with partner**	

Table 9.8: Continued

Summary	Indicators (examples)	Verification (examples)	Assumptions and risks
1.5 Obtain course curriculum and talk to someone who has been to the proposed assertiveness training course to find out more about it	1.5 Discussion with person who has graduated from course	1.5 Feedback form on course completed in positive way	
2.1 Keep a timed activity log of activities at work and outside work	2.1 Completed log by x months demonstrates how time is spent at work and outside work	2.1 Workload log included as underpinning evidence in PDP; activities log reviewed with partner	
2.2 Discuss time/activities log with colleagues at work and family at home. Make plan for non-work activities	2.2 Plan emerged within three months of discussions	2.2 Several colleagues and also your partner at home discuss your log with you; discussion cited in PDP	
2.3 Join a health club and attend induction. Visit several health clubs and try sample days before joining one as member	2.3 Try sample days at two health clubs before joining one as member. Attend induction at health club one week after joining	2.3 Day passes at two health clubs for trials. Membership fee paid; baseline record of fitness completed	
2.4 Review personal and professional diaries and write in non-work activities	2.4 Spaces made in weekly timetable from one month onwards	2.4 Entries for protected time for non-work activities written in diary up to six months ahead	
2.5 Review sources of stress at home from perspectives of self and partner/family and make plans. Discuss stressors and job satisfaction with partner at home	2.5 Draft plan by three months after review	2.5 Draft plan is family document, signed by all	
2.6 Agree a rota with siblings to help parent who is ill	2.6 Agreed rota with siblings for helping parent who is ill	2.6 Entries made on your home calendar for your turn with helping your parent; employ domestic or carer help	

Table 9.8: Continued

Summary	Indicators (examples)	Verification (examples)	Assumptions and risks
2.7 Take up new hobby you have always intended to pursue	2.7 Learn a musical instrument, practise for lessons by x months	2.7 Buy a musical instrument; attend music lessons	
3.1 Convene family meeting to discuss problems and changes everyone wishes to make	3.1 Meeting by x months	3.1 Family meeting convened to discuss review of stress log, problems and solutions, aspirations for change	
3.2 Invite friends round for a series of meals, outings	3.2 Friends invited, time planned in diary	3.2 At least x friends invited to y activities on z occasions	
3.3 Review own and partner's work commitments and career aspirations together	3.3 Met with partner in planned dedicated time when likelihood of interruptions was minimised	3.3 Notes and plan from meeting to obtain further information or advice, or to apply for new posts or training – as relevant	
3.4 Conduct audit of own job satisfaction	3.4 Completed audit of own job satisfaction by x months	3.4 Method of rating job satisfaction shared with partner and others at work	
3.5 Arrangements for meetings with partner and family to discuss changes optimise their attendance (e.g. with dinner or promise of outing afterwards)	3.5 Include outputs of meetings in 3.1 and 3.3 above; summary of positive factors to boost job satisfaction by x months	3.5 Boosting job satisfaction and potential change of work discussed with family and partner at home	

Concluding your logical plan

Now that you have finished mapping out your log frame, you should refine it and discuss it with your partner/spouse or perhaps someone else from outside the family to see whether it is realistic, or whether there is something else that you have not thought of.

Decide how often you are going to review the log frame. A six-monthly review, say, should enable you to keep track of your progress with your project. The extent to which you meet the indicators should give you a good idea of how you are getting on. You may then also realise that there are additional assumptions and risks that you have not previously thought of or addressed.

References

1   Coleman G (1987) Logical framework approach to the monitoring and evaluation of agricultural and rural development projects. *Project Appraisal.* **2**: 251–9.

2   Centre for Rural Development and Training (2000) *A Guide for Developing a Logical Framework.* University of Wolverhampton, Wolverhampton.

3   Jacobs B (2001) *Logical Framework and Performance Management.* North Staffordshire Health Action Zone, Stoke-on-Trent.

4   Spender A and Chambers R (2001) *Logical Framework Plan for Teenwise Project.* Staffordshire University, Stoke-on-Trent (unpublished).

Further reading and audio cassettes about stress and survival matters

Further reading

- Chambers R (2000) *Survival Skills for GPs*. Radcliffe Medical Press, Oxford.
- Cooper CL and Palmer S (2000) *Conquer Your Stress*. Chartered Institute of Personnel and Development, London.
- Cozens J (1991) *OK2 Talk Feelings*. BBC Books, London.
- Denny R (1997) *Succeed for Yourself: unlock your potential for success and happiness*. Kogan Page, London.
- Gillett R (1991) *Overcoming Depression: a practical self-help guide to prevention and treatment*. Dorling Kindersley, London.
- Harris TA (1973) *I'm OK, You're OK*. Pan Books, London.
- Haslam D (ed.) (2000) *Not Another Guide to Stress in General Practice* (2e). Radcliffe Medical Press, Oxford.
- Jeffers S (1987) *Feel the Fear and Do It Anyway*. Rider, London.
- Skynner R and Cleese J (1994) *Families and How to Survive Them*. Mandarin, London.
- Wilkinson G, Moore B and Moore P (2000) *Treating People with Depression. A practical guide for primary care*. Radcliffe Medical Press, Oxford.
- Wilkinson G, Moore B and Moore P (2000) *Treating People with Anxiety and Stress. A practical guide for primary care*. Radcliffe Medical Press, Oxford.
- Woodham A (1995) *Beating Stress at Work*. Health Education Authority, London.

Audio cassettes relating to stress management

Talking Life, 1a Grosvenor Road, Hoylake, Wirral CH47 7BS

Tel: 0151 632 0662 Fax: 0151 632 1206

website: www.talkinglife.co.uk

You can order audio cassettes on *Coping with Stress at Work, Coping with Depression, The Stress Kit, Feeling Good, The Relaxation Kit,* the *Anxiety/Depression Option Pack* and many others, such as Stress Multi Packs and Training Packs (*The Depression Skills Pack, Stress Management Packs, Anxiety and Depression Packs*).

Index